CHILD HEALTH CLINICS

A HANDBOOK
FOR DOCTORS

CHILD HEALTH CLINICS

A HANDBOOK FOR DOCTORS

Margaret Barker MRCP DCH
Consultant Community Paediatrician
West Dorset Health Authority

Jonathan Ferrier MRCGP DRCOG DCH
General Practitioner and
Course Organiser, Oxford

with contributions by
Frances Davies RGN DN HV
Health Visitor
Oxford

JOHN WILEY & SONS

CHICHESTER · NEW YORK · BRISBANE · TORONTO · SINGAPORE

British Library Cataloguing in Publication Data:

Barker, Margaret
  Child health clinics
  1. Pediatric clinics—Great Britain
  I. Title   II. Ferrier, Jonathan   III. Davies, Frances
  362.1'989201'0941   RJ27.5.G7

  ISBN 0 471 91626 9

Library of Congress Cataloging-in-Publication Data:

Barker, Margaret.
  Child health clinics.

  1. Infant health services—Administration—
Handbooks, manuals, etc. 2. Infants—Diseases—
Treatment—Handbooks, manuals, etc. I. Ferrier,
Jonathan.   II. Davies, Frances.   III. Title.
[DNLM: 1. Child Health Services—organization &
administration.   2. Infant Care.   3. Infant, Newborn,
Diseases. WA 320 B255c]
RJ101.B267   1988   618.92   87 – 10487
ISBN 0 471 91626 9 (pbk.)

Typeset by Woodfield Graphics, Fontwell, Arundel, West Sussex.
Printed in Great Britain by Anchor Brendon, Tiptree, Essex.

Contents

PART III—SOCIAL, EMOTIONAL, BEHAVIOURAL PROBLEMS

Preface

This book came to be written because we had each found ourselves in the position of doctor at a well baby clinic with no training that fitted us for the problems we had to face. Neither our student teaching, nor our experience in hospital paediatrics, nor even attendance at courses on developmental paediatrics had adequately prepared us for this work. After learning some of the 'tricks of the trade' the hard way over a number of years, we had both of us started independently to write a practical guide for doctors at these clinics. By coincidence we both approached the same publisher at the same time, and we are very grateful to John Churchill for bringing us together and encouraging us. Further encouragement came from another publisher, Patrick West, who also suggested that we needed an input from a health visitor. Frances Davies agreed to help us and we are greatly indebted to her for the many additions and changes in emphasis that she has been able to bring to the book.

The end result is a book written for doctors, by doctors, with improvements by a health visitor, which we hope will prove of particular interest to G P trainees and Community Medical Officers in training. We also hope that health visitors may find some parts of it relevant to them, although it is not specifically written for them.

It should be obvious that this is intended to be a pocket book that can be easily read from cover to cover in a couple of hours, and which can then be kept handy for immediate reference in a clinic. It should be complementary to the well known paediatric textbooks in which most of the conditions we mention are covered in much greater detail. Our aim has been to describe briefly the common physical and emotional conditions with which patients present in clinics, and to discuss their management. In particular, we try to indicate at what point they should be referred for a specialist opinion, and to give a method of management which we know works from our own experience.

Although it would be inappropriate for a new doctor at a clinic to make immediate changes, we feel that it is important for him to know how a clinic should function and about its place in prevention, education and developmental checks. We have covered this in the first section of the book.

MARGARET BARKER
JONATHAN FERRIER
1987

Acknowledgements

We are very much in the debt of a surprisingly large number of people considering the size of this book. Perhaps it is a measure of how little has been written on this subject, that we should have needed to ask so many questions but we certainly required and are grateful for the help of the following:

Mr Michael Benson—Consultant Orthopaedic Surgeon, Oxford.
Mr Graham Hall—Consultant Orthopaedic Surgeon, West Dorset.
Mr Malcolm Gough—Consultant Surgeon, Oxford.
Mr Michael Poole—Consultant Plastic Surgeon, Oxford.
Dr Inga Ostman-Smith—Consultant Paediatric Cardiologist, Oxford.
Dr Richard Purvis—Consultant Paediatrician, West Dorset.
Mrs Sue Chapman for the colour photographs.
Mrs Joan Jeffries, Mrs Carole Close and Mrs Judith Douglas for the typing.
The Department of Medical Illustration, Oxford, for the black and white photographs and the art work.

We should like to thank Mr and Mrs Lee for the picture of their 'young professionals' on the front cover and all the other parents who kindly allowed us to photograph their children.

Finally, we should like to dedicate this book to our own children (all 9 of them) who taught us more about childhood than anyone else, and usually the hard way.

Part I

THE NORMAL CLINIC

1

Introduction

WHAT IT'S ABOUT

We have had to find for ourselves the answers to many of the problems that face us in child health clinics and have set these down. Many such issues have no definitive management and ours are by no means the only solutions. They may not even always be the best ones and we would like to hear from anyone with more effective suggestions. However, we hope that we have managed to include most of the common problems ranging from those of organisation, through physical conditions, to emotional and behavioural disorders.

We have not covered developmental assessment in the sort of detail that some experts in this field use routinely because we feel that such an approach is not practicable in a busy clinic. We try to use a few, quick simple tests to confirm that development is within the normal range and then spend as much time as possible discussing the parents' queries with them, whether they are about general management of their children or specific worries. Further detailed assessment or investigation is then arranged if necessary.

WHO IT'S FOR

It can be alarming to the young doctor recently out of hospital to start work in a child health clinic and find himself suddenly expected to answer questions which he has never met before. They will be about children who are not ill but are worrying their parents, and he will be expected to give answers confidently and competently. He must know when to reassure, how to give guidance and when to refer for a further opinion.

Many child health clinics are now being run with general practitioners as the clinic doctors, and it is likely that this trend will increase. Yet GPs have mainly had experience of ill children in busy surgeries or hospital wards, and may have little concept of what is expected of them in a clinic for well babies, nor of what can potentially be achieved there. Furthermore, some doctors dislike these clinics, and we suspect this is partly because they feel unsure of what they should be doing in them, and partly because they feel they could be spending their time better elsewhere. We hope we have offered some answers here and in particular we hope this will be of use to GP trainees.

3

Health visitors have a well-established training which includes practical guidance, but the newly-qualified health visitor still has to face the early sessions when she first copes alone in a child health clinic. Many of the questions she is asked will be the same as those asked of the doctor, but she has the added decision to make of whether a child needs a further assessment by a doctor. We think that if she has a reasonable idea of when a physical condition is likely to need referral and how a management problem can be approached, she will have a good basis from which to start.

WHO'S WHO

After some debate between ourselves, we agreed that all doctors should be referred to as he, health visitors and parents as she, and children as he, except for specifically female conditions. We are fully aware that half the doctors and children are female, and while we are still waiting to meet our first male health visitor, we have noticed that children are not infrequently these days brought to the clinics by their fathers. However, we felt we should risk the wrath of some sections of society in the interests of clarity and trying to make our text more readable.

To our way of thinking, the terms Well Baby Clinic and Child Health Clinic are synonymous and are used indiscriminately throughout the book.

2

The Organisation of a
Child Health Clinic

The child health clinic is a well baby clinic, forming a major part of the child
health service. It is a service for well children from birth to school age, their
parents and/or their carers.

The activities of a child health clinic may be considered as follows:

1 giving information, advice, support, reassurance, counselling (see Chap-
   ters 11 – 14)
2 developmental surveillance (see Chapter 4)
3 developmental screening programmes (see Chapter 4)
4 immunisation (see Chapter 5)
5 health education,
6 socialisation among the parents, carers, children and the clinic team.

How these activities are organised within the clinic will vary from district
to district. The needs of the local clients should be taken into consideration
with regard to day and time of the clinic: for example, evening clinics may
be appreciated; 'drop-in' clinics may be more useful than those with appointment systems; immunisation-only clinics, with booked appointments, may be
needed.

PREMISES

The provision of premises which are easily accessible to the clients have been
found to be more important than the quality of the clinic building. However,
it is useful to consider some of the basic needs of clinic premises:

1 car-parking and covered pram-parking facilities,
2 rooms which are welcoming, bright and clean,
3 adequate warmth and lighting,
4 main social waiting and play area,
5 facilities for private consultation with doctor and health visitor,
6 facilities for private developmental screening, surveillance, and
   immunisation procedures,
7 facilities for feeding and changing babies.

The ideal child health clinic is situated in the ground floor of a building
which is reasonably central to the area it covers.

The waiting room needs to be large enough for the mothers not to be crowded together, and to allow an area for helpers to keep a register and weigh the babies. Equally, it should not feel like an aircraft hangar!

For choice, there should also be three separate smaller rooms for the doctor, health visitor and nurse. The doctor and health visitor each need a room with facilities for consulting with the mothers, examining the babies and children and hand washing. It is preferable for the immunisation injections to be given in a separate room by the clinic nurse, although in the smaller clinics these are often given by the doctor or the health visitor.

Altogether, these facilities are most likely to be found in a purpose-built surgery or health centre, although a converted house can be every bit as well laid out, and may seem to be a great deal less clinical. On the other hand, some designers of surgeries seem to have forgotten entirely about child health clinics in their planning, with a waiting room that is too small and with the health visitor banished to a dowdy council office half a mile away.

THE TEAM

The team which works within the child health clinic may vary in its composition, but all members should have specific training and commitment to child health. This underlines the need for multidisciplinary training and role appreciation (ie. understanding what the other members of the team are trained to do, and why), particularly between the health visitor and the clinic doctor. The health visitor has to have easy access to expert medical opinion and, conversely, the clinic doctor should be able to discuss feeding, behavioural management and social problems with the health visitor. It is essential that frequent discussion should take place between the members of the team to ensure that parents do not receive conflicting advice.

The parent or carer of the child should feel able to draw freely upon the expertise available within the team.

The Health Visitor

The health visitor is the key person in a child health clinic. She has to organise the clinic and act as the liaison between all the people who run it but, more importantly, she is the contact with the families in their homes. Her personality and approach to the job is therefore all-important, and it is essential that she should come across as a warm, friendly and approachable person while providing an efficient service.

Her first contact with the parents is usually at the antenatal (parentcraft) classes, so that she is already recognised as someone who can offer support before the baby is even born, and the parents know how she will be able to help them in the future. It can be an enormous relief for a mother to have a knowledgeable, friendly health visitor whom she knows will be available to counsel and advise her. This particularly applies to mothers who are breast feeding for the first time, and to mothers who might be expected to 'know it all', such as doctors, nurses and health visitors.

Further contact will mostly take place at the well baby clinic sessions but as these are held only once a week, at most, it is therefore essential that a health visitor should be available at other times. One way to achieve this is for the health visitor to have her own direct line and let it be known that she will always be in her office for calls between 0900 and 1000 on weekdays.

There are considerable advantages when that office is part of the GPs' surgery. Experienced reception staff may spot families with problems as soon as they register and they, or the doctor, can immediately alert the health visitor. Likewise, the best follow-up for such events as a cot death, or a child diagnosed as having a malignancy or mental retardation, can be organised if the GP can liaise easily with health visitor and discuss the problems as they arise. The feedback will also work the other way: for example, the health visitor will often be the first to pick up postnatal depression, or the baby who at first appears to have a feeding problem, but then turns out to have a more serious condition such as heart disease.

The Doctor

Doctors have a slightly different role in child health clinics compared with a GP's surgery. The health visitor has the overall responsibility for organising the clinic, which means that the doctor's most important function is to provide medical back-up and expertise. It is therefore important that the doctor actually does know the answers to many of the problems which are brought to him. It is interesting to see how pleased parents are when they discover that the doctor has children of his own. They rightly feel that many of the things that worry them are simply part of everyday life, and can be simply answered by someone who has experience of bringing up a family. It is, however, incumbent on the doctor to know not only about everyday matters such as feeding problems, but also the point at which minor symptoms should be taken more seriously and referred elsewhere.

It is often preferable that the clinic doctor should be the patient's own GP, because he will know the background of the whole family and will usually have established a relationship with the mother. He is also likely to be looking after the child in sickness as well as at clinic attendances, so that he has every opportunity to get to know the child and establish a good rapport. However, he must have the basic knowledge mentioned above and, even more importantly, he must be interested in the welfare of the children. It is far better that the clinic doctor should be a clinical medical officer from the community who is interested in the children than a disinterested GP who has been pushed into the job against his wishes.

Clinical Medical Officers (or Community Child Health Doctors) have until recently been the only doctors in child health clinics. Their original function there, as a separate group of doctors employed by the local authority, was to fill an urgent need for examining and treating children whose families were too poor to attend a doctor except in extreme illness. This important role declined once the National Health Service was established, but in the past decade the more senior of these doctors have evolved as specialists in developmental and educational paediatrics. It is likely that this trend towards specialist level will continue as, increasingly, health visitors and GPs take responsibility for the primary screening of young children, but at present there is an interim situation of great variety. This flexible variety seems to us desirable if it ensures that the doctor who attends each clinic is the one most interested in it.

The Nurse

Some of the larger child health clinics have a nurse attached, employed by the health authority. Where there are large numbers of children for injection her presence can be invaluable because she will free the health visitor and doctor to spend more time with the patients. However, giving injections is by no means her only function: she can help with testing hearing, pre-school checks and many other procedures. She may be the school nurse for a number of primary schools in the area of the clinic, and in this case she will provide a most valuable link between school and clinic.

Where the clinic is held in a doctor's surgery and no local authority nurse is supplied, a practice nurse may be able to help. In this case, the GP can claim the injection fees under form FP73 which will therefore pay the cost of employing her for that session. While the links with the school will not be made, her greater involvement with the families will be a help in the practice, because at times of illness the mothers will feel they know the surgery staff, and the nurse herself may have useful background information to pass on to the doctor.

PROBLEMS

Access

Problems may arise in child health clinics from the fact that most clinics run on an open access system, so that anyone who turns up will be seen. This invariably means that on some days there will be very few patients, while on others staff are run off their feet with the consequence that the mothers may not get enough time to mention their real worries. To some extent, with experience, one can predict the busy clinics (for instance, the first one after term has started), but even then one may be proved wrong and in any case will probably be unable to increase staffing.

We feel strongly that open access is an important principle to maintain, because it allows the mother to come at the time she needs help. It is therefore necessary to even out the workload and this can most easily be done by issuing appointments for the routine work of immunisations and health checks, leaving enough time for the 'drop-ins'. Appointments for health checks will usually be made by the health visitor, while those for immunisation may originate from a central computer.

Workload

Sometimes the workload turns out to be unequal between the different members of the team, leaving one person in a frantic rush while another has nothing to do, but with goodwill this situation should not arise. There really is no need for rigid job discrimination. Of course, there may be some things that can only be done by the doctor (eg. checking the heart), and others that are usually dealt with by the health visitor (eg. routine feeding advice), but many things can be done equally well by either of them, such as the 18-month and three-year checks.

GP practice business and visits should become the responsibility of another GP in the group during the time the doctor is working within the Clinic.

Records

Record cards in child health clinics are usually provided by the health authority and kept by the health visitor responsible for each clinic. Every health authority in Britain seems to have its own clinic card, which varies from the immensely detailed to what is virtually a blank sheet of paper. Some authorities are now experimenting with cards which are kept by the patients (or at least their parents) which will presumably have certain advantages and disadvantages. It would really simplify matters if there was a standard card for use throughout the country, with a duplicate portion of certain parts to be kept by the family.

The fundamental requirements for recording are:

Names	Immunisations
Date of birth	Birth history
Sex	Basic checks
Address	Percentile charts of weight,
Siblings	Height, head circumference

If too much detail is included, it becomes impossible to find the important information, and the process of recording becomes a meaningless list of ticks. Where no information is specifically requested, an examiner at a later date has no idea what has been checked, ie. does 'NAD' mean 'Nothing Abnormal Discovered' or 'Not Actually Done'?

3

Examining Children

You will probably have come across two sorts of doctor who show extremes of good and bad examination technique with children. There is the one for whom all children behave like angels; to an adult they may seem rather severe but children come up to them and perform as if trained to do so, whilst plainly enjoying the experience. Then there is the doctor whose abruptness and off-handedness can reduce the most self-composed child to tears. Most of us fall between the two, but with practice we can improve our technique to obtain a rapport with the great majority of our patients. We have therefore included this chapter to give a few suggestions which may be helpful.

THE SET-UP

Children under four (and sometimes over) are best seen sitting on their mother's knee beside the doctor—this brings them to the same height as the doctor and gives them the security they need to allow themselves to be examined. Every now and then you will have a parent who tells her three or four-year-old to 'sit down beside the doctor', walks to the side of the room, and then says to the child 'Tell the doctor what's wrong'. No wonder the poor thing looks bewildered. Other parents get into a terrible state worrying that their child will behave badly. They keep telling the child that 'the doctor is not going to hurt you' which in effect tells the child that this is a possibility, when he probably would never have considered it. Some parents keep trying desperately to distract their child's attention, eg. 'Look at that picture on the wall', 'What's that outside the window?', which again indicates to him that the stethoscope or the auriscope, or the doctor himself, are all too terrible to look at. Luckily, the children of such parents know them only too well, and resolutely ignore such trivia—they either look the doctor full in the face or bury their heads.

With children over four, their best co-operation will usually be obtained if they stand by their parent's knee while the parent sits beside the doctor's desk. Again, they will feel deserted if you allow the parent to sit away from the child.

When there are two or more children to be seen, it is generally best to start with the child who is likely to behave best, remembering that 18 months is about the worst age for co-operation. Under one year of age, most children

10

will accept anyone new but after about two years they become increasingly good at summing up the situation and deciding that nobody is going to hurt them. However, many children in their second year look on all strangers as capable of major assault and have their worst fears confirmed when the doctor looms over them with a stethoscope. For this reason a useful approach is often to welcome the mother into the room, say 'hello' to the child and then ignore him completely while you talk to the mother. This gives him time to assess you and the surroundings, and he will also pick up the fact that his mother is not afraid of you.

If he has come for a routine check, the child's confidence can be increased by offering him something simple to play with, such as a brick for an eight-month-old, or several bricks and a plastic beaker at 18 months. However, if you engage his full attention with a really interesting toy, such as a car, you will not be able to get his attention back later and may have screams when you want to take it from him.

If you want to make a physical examination it is obvious that you should start with the least threatening part of it. In any sick child the triad of chest (heart), ears and throat is mandatory and it is usually best to make the examination in that sequence. (Although there should be a firm policy of not seeing sick children at child health clinics, in practice there will be times when you feel obliged to do so.)

EXAMINING THE CHEST AND HEART

When examining a young child with a stethoscope, it is essential not to move too fast or to tower over him. After asking the mother to pull up his clothing (but not over his face!) show him the end of your stethoscope and then slowly put it on his chest. You will at this point be leaning forward so that you are on the same height as the child. If the child is wriggling you may be able to settle him by looking him straight in the eye, or by gently holding one of his hands.

With a child who may be ill, it is often useful to check the pulse, which is most easily done by listening to the pulse rather than trying to palpate it at the wrist. It is worth remembering that a resting pulse in a healthy child is usually about 120 per minute until the age of 12 to 15 months when it falls to about 80. Where the heart rate is very rapid it is possible to count it by starting again every five seconds: in this way you can count up to 15 beats in five seconds which, of course, is a rate of 180.

Even the most perfectly-behaved young child will not sit still for ever, so do not jeopardise your rapport by spending five minutes listening to the heart. Try and get the information you want (heart rate and murmurs) in 30 seconds, and then move to the chest. If you hear a murmur you can come back to it when you have completed the rest of your examination.

A quick listen to both apices of the chest will often suffice in a well child, but if you think there may be something wrong, then you can best hear the bases by sitting the child sideways on his mother's knee.

Some children hold their breath when you touch them with a stethoscope. For the young ones it is probably better simply to wait rather than exhort them to take deep breaths, because the longer they hold their breath, the more deeply will they breathe in the end. However, older children will copy you perfectly (much better than adults) if you demonstrate the way you wish them to breathe.

EXAMINING THE EARS

For Earache

If a child has complained of earache, it is well worth asking him (not the parent) 'Which ear hurts?'. When there is a true otitis media he will unhesitatingly point to the affected ear, but when he seems uncertain you will probably find nothing, or only an exudate behind the tympanic membranes (occasionally, of course, a child will be found to have severe otitis media in both ears at the same time). You should then look in the good ear first, for two reasons; it gives you a baseline for assessing the bad ear, and if the drum has perforated or there is an otitis externa, you will not transfer the infection to the good ear.

When examining the ears of a child who is sitting on his mother's lap, you will find it easiest if she turns him sideways so that she can hold his head still against her chest with one hand. Her other hand can be placed on his arm and shoulder to hold him against her, restraining his arm at the same time. Mothers usually do this naturally, but they commonly make the mistake of covering the child's face with the hand which is holding his head, with the result that not only can he not see what is happening, but he is half-suffocated as well. No child will tolerate this for long, so before you start to look in the ear get her to change hands so that he is held still but can clearly see what you are doing.

A useful trick is then to turn on your auriscope before you fit the plastic speculum and show it to the child. He can then see that it is only a light and not in any way likely to be painful.

For Deafness

The parents' comments about hearing should be listened to with great care. When a mother says that she wonders whether her child is hearing properly, you will need to check the following points:

History: Does he only hear what he wishes, or does he appear not to hear even when he is paying attention, eg. does he sit near the TV and keep turning up the volume? Does he fail to hear any mention of sweets, etc? Family history, past medical history and speech may also be relevant.

Examination: Normal tympanic membranes with an insignificant amount of wax look pearly-coloured and clearly translucent. Opacity, in-drawing or air bubbles are abnormal, although the last may indicate that the middle ear is about to clear.

Hearing test: See Chapter 4.

EXAMINING THE THROAT

No child actually enjoys having his throat examined but with good technique you can make the experience brief and painfree. A young child should be sitting well back on his mother's lap and facing forwards. She can then put one arm across his chest to restrain both his body and his arms and hold his head still and slightly tilted back with the other hand so that it rests against her chest. Do not let her (a) try and hold him while her hands are full of tissues, toys, etc., or (b) try to force his mouth open herself.

Some children will open their mouth when asked to do so, and you may only need to depress the tongue slightly to see the tonsils and pharynx. In this case, let him see your tongue depressor, say 'I'm going to touch your tongue' and do exactly that. (Do not say 'I am going to look at your throat', which makes anyone gag at the mere suggestion.) Very occasionally, a child will open his mouth so wide that you do not even need to depress the tongue.

The majority of very young children will not open their mouth when asked. In this case slip the tongue depressor down the side of the mouth outside the teeth and press it against the teeth. The child will then open his mouth and you can quickly slide it onto the tongue. Provided you are ready with your light pointing in the right direction, his head tilted correctly, and your eyes at the right level, you will see all you need in the next second, and the whole procedure will be over before he even has time to gag.

With a child over the age of four, the use of a tongue depressor can often be avoided by asking him to 'pant like a dog'.

SUMMARY OF EXAMINATION TECHNIQUES

Check chest, ears, throat in that order

1	Chest	— Show stethoscope
		— Listen to pulse, heart sounds, both lungs anteriorly
		— Listen to back, if necessary
2	Ears	— Sit child sideways on mother's lap
		— Hold firmly, not covering the face,
		— Show auriscope
		— Examine good ear first.
3	Throat	— Sit child well back on mother's lap
		— Arms, body and head held firmly
		— Show tongue depressor
		— Ask child to open mouth
		— Insert tongue depressor

4

Developmental Screening

Developmental screening compares each child's development with that of a large sample of normal children of the same age, race and culture. It involves a small number of standardised tests and not necessarily a medical examination, but demands sound knowledge and experience of the range of normal development.
Developmental assessment is a more detailed working-out of the level which a retarded child has reached and it is considered to be a specialised skill. Children whose developmental screening tests are unsatisfactory should be referred for specialist assessment, according to local arrangements.
Developmental surveillance is a term used to cover all the contacts made between the child health professionals and each child which adds up to an overall picture of his progress. Since it also includes the prevention of disease (by immunisation and health education) it is better termed 'health surveillance'.

The remainder of this chapter is about developmental screening. There are no specific ages at which everyone agrees that screening should take place and many different age programmes are in use throughout the country. The only important factor affecting an age choice is that some testable milestones are reached by the majority of normal children at that age. *The Court Report's recommendation for a minimum screening programme is*:

(a) At birth
(b) 6 – 10 days } medical examination done by a doctor with paediatric experience.

(c) 6 weeks — predominantly medical examination but vision, hearing and maturing nervous system can be tested. Done by paediatrically experienced doctor or specially trained health visitor.

(d) 7 – 8 months
(e) 18 months } developmental screening done by health visitor.

(f) 2½ – 3 years — developmental screening done by health visitor plus, if possible, medical examination by doctor.

Most districts employ a programme something like this, and research is in progress to assess the effectiveness of screening at various ages, using a variety of tests, with the aim of defining an optimum system.

14

DECIDING ON WHICH TESTS TO USE

There are as many different schedules of tests as there are programmes for the ages being tested. It is clear that measurements of growth and tests of vision and hearing must be included in some of the screening contacts you have with the child, but which need to be included when? There are certain points which are important in choosing a developmental test:

1   Each test should have a defined progression of stages or a set cut-off point which has been proved in large numbers of normal children of similar culture to those you are testing.
2   Each test should cover only one or two spheres of development (ie. hearing, or speech or movement, etc.) although there is usually a certain amount of overlap—eg. the turning response to sound tests hearing but is dependent on the baby having adequate vision.
3   Each test should be easy and quick to perform, using a minimum of equipment, and should have some element of fun for the child, his parent and the examiner.
4   The tests should be used repeatedly by the same examiner, keeping the number of them to a minimum so that any variation from normal in a child's response is spotted immediately.
5   Certain tests are essential at certain ages because of their major significance, eg. head circumference in the first year of life, squint test by 8 – 10 months, hearing by 10 months.

A suggested schedule is given at the end of this chapter.

OBSERVATION AND HISTORY-TAKING

Observation and history-taking are an essential part of screening. Developmental screening is not simply a quick series of mechanical tests but depends just as much on experienced observation of the child and relevant history-taking. The points which should particularly be observed are:

    Alertness
    Activity
    Attention span
    Ability to relate positively or negatively to a stranger or near-stranger.
and   Attitude to the family, especially his mother, eg. clinging, affectionate, moves away readily, etc. or to siblings, eg. dominated by older sister, attacks baby, etc.

The history must include brief details of delivery, early milestones, illnesses, and so on, but if a continuous recording system is kept these facts will already be to hand. Matters related to the child's family and environment will also be relevant.

MEASUREMENTS

Weight

A child's weight is an obvious indicator of his growth but there was a phase in child health clinics for it to be the only indicator that was measured and this has left a legacy of public opinion that thinks the only reason for taking a child to a clinic is to plonk him on the scales. As a reaction against this there has recently been a tendency in professional journals and elsewhere to criticise any frequent weighing of a baby. There must be a commonsense path between these two extremes and our choice is to aim for enough accurate weights for a percentile chart to have validity. This generally means that we try to obtain a naked weight (either by weighing a naked baby or, if the environment is quite unsuited to this, by weighing in minimum clothing which has been taken into account) as often as fortnightly until four to six months of age and then at each developmental screening contact. All these weights must be entered on to a percentile chart.

For those who are unfamiliar with using *percentile charts*, a brief explanation will be given. These are straightforward graphs of weight or height or head circumference (or any other measureable attainment) plotted against age, but they have the added bonus of showing the curve that is followed by children growing 'normally'—called the 50th percentile because, at any point on that curve, 50% of children at that age will weigh less than that amount. Each side of this curve are others, up to the 97th percentile (at any point on this curve 97% of children of that age will be less than that weight) and down to the third percentile. These represent ± 2 standard deviations so that, if a child's personal weight curve is below the third percentile or above the 97th percentile, it is significantly different from the rest of the childhood population and needs due consideration. Perhaps more important still is the child whose weight curve starts off near to one percentile line then flattens off or descends to join another one or cross several (see Figures 4.1a–d). This gives a prompt indication that something may be going wrong for that child and more investigation of his eating, health and circumstances are needed. A single weight can only give this sort of important information if previous accurate weights of a child are available and plotted on a chart.

Height

It has become essential in recent years to make an early diagnosis in any child with growth hormone deficiency if he is to benefit fully from the expensive treatment that is now available. Short stature does not become obvious to parents until their child mixes with others of the same age, usually not until he is five or six years of age. It should therefore be actively looked for by screening all children for height deficiency. A single measurement of height is insufficient and at least two measurements about six months apart are necessary to say that a child is not only short but is growing very slowly. Screening measurements of height, which will pick out the children who need this follow-up, can conveniently be done at the time of other screening tests.

In the first year of life the only accurate way to measure length is with a special board (plastic portable versions are now available). This entails laying the baby on his back with his head touching a head-board, then a foot-board is placed against his soles, fixed in position, the baby removed and the distance between the two boards measured. It is obvious, if you try this, that at least two pairs of hands are needed and, even then, a crying baby is liable to flex his hips and knees and make an accurate measurement nearly impossible.

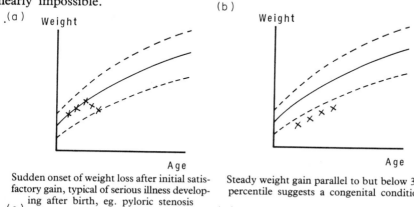

(a) Weight / Age
Sudden onset of weight loss after initial satisfactory gain, typical of serious illness developing after birth, eg. pyloric stenosis

(b) Weight / Age
Steady weight gain parallel to but below 3rd percentile suggests a congenital condition

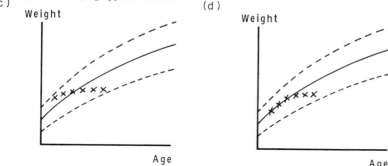

(c) Weight / Age
Failure of a large baby who was normal at birth to gain weight suggests feeding problems or, more rarely, a malabsorption condition

(d) Weight / Age
Levelling-out of weight gain, possibly due to illness or inadequate feeding

Fig 4.1   Unsatisfactory weight charts

Beyond 18 months Once the child can stand and straighten his knees with his feet together, any conventional height measure can be used. It is essential that the child's heels are together against the measure and his head held up by lifting under the angles of his jaw. If standard equipment is not available the measurement can be made against a wall provided care is taken to ensure accuracy.

All height measurements are only meaningful when plotted on a percentile chart. If a child's growth curve is persistently below the 3rd percentile, he should have some investigations done and therefore needs referral. The cause may well be familial but this must not be assumed to be so until other causes have been eliminated, since some of these are also familial but potentially treatable. This referral should be done before the child is of school age.

Head Circumference

This is difficult to do accurately and varies considerably from one observer to another. There are accurate portable measures available but most of us use only a tape measure. This should be of firm plastic or paper, not cloth, so that it is not stretchy. A measurement at birth may be of little significance because of moulding but a measurement within the first week is essential as a first point on a percentile chart. Repeat measurements should be made at each developmental check up to 18 months of age and the resulting curve on a percentile chart clearly indicates which children need further investigation of their development, family head size, or skull, brain and ventricular growth.

HEARING AND VISION TESTS

Hearing

This is a very important part of developmental testing, not only because of the need to institute proper management of a deaf child but also because his deafness will affect the whole of his development and behaviour. There are specialised tests available from a very early age for any child if there is doubt about his hearing in the early weeks or months of life, and referral to a suitable department should not be delayed.

At the six-to-eight week check testing is crude and only shows that the auditory pathways are probably intact. It is more important to ask the mother if she thinks her baby can hear. A sudden sound (eg. a clap) should produce a sharp blink of the baby's eyes and shaking a bell or rattle out of his field of vision should cause him to be still for a second. Care must be taken not to create a draught when clapping nor a vibration such as banging the examination couch.

At the seven-to-nine month age group distraction testing can be quite accurately and easily done. It should be taught to every clinic doctor and health visitor individually.

The child sits on his mother's lap, at the edge of her knees, and faces forward to the person who is going to distract, ie. quietly and with minimum activity draw the child's attention towards her. The tester stands behind mother and baby and makes a short series of high-pitched and low-pitched sounds at minimal volume, on a level with each of the child's ears (see diagram for positions). To each of these sounds the baby should turn round. The sounds are:

— a soft (40dB or less) 'ooh' in a low voice;
— a soft (40dB or less) 'sss' or 'ttt' (as in it, not tub);

— gently turning a special high-tone rattle;
— (others, such as tissue paper rattling, spoon touching cup edge, from the Stycar test of hearing are open to careless use at far too loud a level and should not be used);
— (if available, a 'Warbler'—a hand-held little instrument that produces an interesting sound at fixed frequency levels, which is really more accurate than the voice but does not always seem as interesting to a baby as to older children).

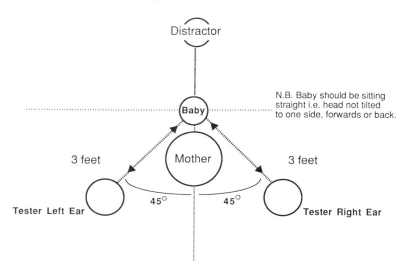

Fig 4.2   Distraction testing for hearing ability

Essential points to note to avoid errors in distraction testing are:

— the child's vision must be adequate for him to have learnt that sounds come from a source;
— sounds must be made on a level with the child's ear because he cannot at this age locate them above or below his ear-level;
— the tester must not give any visual clue to the child or create a draught. Mirrors or glass in front of the child can be a particular source of falsely normal results—deaf children are very visually aware;
— the volume of sound must be kept very soft—practising this with a sound-level indicator is the best way of learning to keep the volume below 40dB, but if one is not available practise making the sounds at the quietest 'ordinary' voice that you can achieve, ie. not a whisper;
— the tester must have normal hearing, otherwise the sounds will be made too loudly;
— a child aged less than six months or more than about 12 months is not reliably tested by this method, the younger ones because they have not learnt to locate sound sources, and the older ones because

they will choose whether or not they turn to look for a sound;
— the developmentally-delayed child may not have reached a six-month level and so will 'fail' the test—parents will thus begin to believe him to be deaf rather than slow. Prompt referral to a developmental assessment clinic, if he is not already attending one, is necessary. If the developmental delay is already known, it is better to avoid doing a routine hearing test, provided the paediatrician looking after the child is informed so that he can arrange more appropriate testing. The child with a physical handicap may also be unable to do a distraction hearing test because of poor head-control.

In older children. Few tests are very satisfactory between the ages of one year and about 2¼ years and real doubt about hearing in this age-group warrants referral to a specialist department. From 2¼ to 2½ years onwards performance tests can be used. There are a number of these available—Nottingham toy test, Stycar test, Michael Reed cards, Manchester test, free-field audiometry, etc.—and each has its own set of instructions. None is a total test of all aspects of the ability to hear but any can be used as a screening test. Younger children co-operate best with a toy test, in which they are asked, in a quiet voice and avoiding the possibility of lip reading, to indicate individual toys from a group that have similar-sounding names (eg. duck, cup; tree, key, etc.) Children of 3½ years or more can use picture tests, which are similar but quicker to use, or they can carry out tests which involve doing something (for example, putting a brick into a box) each time they hear a sound from a Warbler or free-field audiometer. Once a child is reliably co-operative in these tasks, he can manage to use head-phones and a pure-tone audiometer and an accurate measurement of hearing can be made.

Tympanography can be very useful even in young children but is not generally available in clinics.

Whatever a child's age, a failed hearing test should lead on to a proper procedure of follow-up and this is discussed further in Chapter 10.

Vision

Any child's development will be hampered if he does not see himself, his family and his environment clearly. There are objective tests of vision which require specialist skills and work is always in process to find new screening methods which are more objective than the existing ones, but at present the following fairly crude tests are in use:-

At six to eight weeks of age a baby's mother can usually tell you if her child can see. He should certainly be able to smile at her and his vision can be tested by drawing his attention to an alternative object (eg. a red ball—or the examiner's face!) held about 12 inches from his eyes then watching him follow it through an arc of 180° in each direction. If he is crying or his eyes remain firmly shut, a successful examination may still be achieved by asking his mother to hold him so that he looks over her shoulder. Often, the baby will then open his eyes and, by standing behind the mother, you can continue your examination. A brief look at each eye with an ophthalmoscope to see the 'red reflex' confirms that no congenital cataract is present.

At six months or more, routine testing may only consist of checking for squint by the asymmetry that a squint produces when a light is reflected in the cornea, and by a 'cover test', which should pick up even a latent squint (see Chapter 7).

At nine months or more there are a few tests which attempt to assess visual acuity but only the fixed-ball test of the Stycar kit is accurate and it really is not practicable as a portable screening test.

From three years onwards, visual acuity can be measured with some accuracy by a matching test in which the child has either a key-card of letters or pictures or else solid plastic letters or even a set of toys (Stycar test) whilst the examiner has the equivalent letters, pictures or toys in a graded series of diminishing size. These are shown to the child from a fixed distance, usually three metres, saying 'Show me the one that looks like this'. Each test kit that is available has its own instructions but all are based on the same principle. It is essential to continue with the test until each of the child's eyes has been tested separately, if necessary repeating the test on one or two later occasions, since the main purpose of screening vision at this young age is to pick up any child in danger of developing amblyopia.

Two useful points about these tests are:
— a plastic 'pirate patch' or a wooden or plastic spoon is tolerated better for occluding one eye than an adult's hand;
— if a child is totally co-operative for testing one eye but gets upset quickly for the other, your suspicions should be aroused that he has very poor vision in that eye. After a few minutes break, try the test again, starting with the 'difficult' eye. If the result is the same, it is wiser promptly to refer the child to a specialist department than to presume that he is being difficult and recall him.

At five years of age, children need a visual acuity good enough to allow them to scan letters in a line, so testing must be done with a wall-chart, well illuminated at six metres distance. A key-card of the letters for matching can be used if they cannot be reliably named and, again, each eye must be tested separately.

Referral of children who have had unsatisfactory vision tests should be to an ophthalmologist, according to local arrangements, and this is mentioned again in Chapter 10.

TESTS OF MANIPULATION
(and their use to demonstrate other skills)
Using Small Bricks.

Textbook descriptions of these tests all use one-inch coloured wooden cubes, but these are not easy to obtain and there is no harm in settling for some variation on this which can be bought at the local toy shop. Give them a thorough wash in warm water when newly bought, so that any colour which is going to come out does so there rather than on your first patient's lips and clothes! There is a recognised series of normal activities which babies carry out when presented with such bricks but only a few stages will be described here.

By eight months a baby will pick up a brick using a palmar (whole-hand) grasp, take it to his mouth and change hands with it, both hands then being at his midline. If another brick is offered, he will open his hand and discard the held brick without looking at it.

At nine months he can pick a brick up in each hand, using a 'coarse pincer' grip, ie. two fingers and thumb in apposition, and will look at the bricks before mouthing them.

At 18 months he can pile three or four bricks into a tower, has ceased mouthing and does not discard them blindly on to the floor. He can post them into a container and lift them back out and, if you cover a brick with the container he will instantly lift the cover and look for the hidden brick. He is also likely to demonstrate that he can throw them forwards, although this is obviously preferably tested with a soft ball!

At three years he will build more bricks, provided the surface is stable enough, and will make a 'bridge' of three bricks if you show him how, even if you knock your model over or cover it up. During this year of life he will learn to match the coloured bricks, if you say 'Find me a brick that looks just like this', and he will demonstrate the use of 3 prepositions 'Put the brick in/on/under the box'. If your bricks have a hole drilled smoothly through them, he will thread them on to a stiff piece of nylon but, of course, beads which can easily be gripped are just as good. If you store the bricks in a screw-top jar, he will also demonstrate that he can unscrew the top.

At four to five years he will copy more complicated models made with the bricks, of which the classical ones are a gate made with five bricks and stairs made with six, but there is no fixed time during this year of age when these skills are achieved. He knows at least one more preposition and can name colours, provided somebody has taught him their names.

Using a Pencil and Paper.

This does not become useful as a screening test until 18 months of age. At that stage a child will hold the end of the pencil furthest from the lead in a whole-hand grasp and make a few tentative scribble strokes on the paper before he becomes distracted on to seeing what else he can do with it. It should form only a brief part of a screening test at this age and perhaps erves more as a reminder to parents that the child needs some experience of drawing than as a test of any significance.

At *two years* his scribble marks will be more confident and confluent and may be back-and-forth lines or round-and-round sweeps. He may be quite difficult to divert from this activity but you will notice him changing hands with the pencil, often as he reaches his own midline.

At *three years* he can readily take the pencil off the page to make discrete marks and his grip will be near the point but not necessarily a tripod grasp. He will be able to draw a cross and circle if you do them first for him. He may be developing a clear preference for one hand but may still change over at times.

At *four to five years* he should have a tripod grasp of the pencil, ie. two fingers and thumb, but it will be rigid rather than the mobile flexing of finger-joints of an older child or adult. He will copy a circle and cross, and attempt a square, although this may only have one angled corner at first and otherwise looks like a circle. He should have a definite preference for one hand but will sometimes draw a picture upside down or sideways without apparently noticing the difference.

Drawing a man

This can be a formalised test from about three years onwards, with scores worked out from the amount of detail spontaneously included (called the Goodenough Draw-a-man Test). It is useful as part of a developmental assessment but is unnecessary in screening. However, to ask a child of three years and over to draw a face or a man may give ample opportunity for hearing his speech and testing his understanding, and certainly adds greatly to the entertainment value of the test without taking too much time. It can also form a useful baseline for comparison with any subsequent screening or formal testing done in his early school years.
For brief TESTS OF LANGUAGE see chapter 10, pages 70 – 71.

EQUIPMENT

It should now be evident that the essential tests of development in the pre-school child can be carried out with a minimum of equipment and cost. A suggested basic kit can consist of:

— a tape measure (not cloth) and percentile charts
— access to an accurate weighing scales
— a high-tone rattle and/or warbler
— a performance test of hearing—one test with toys and, optionally, a picture test
— 10 small bricks, with at least two of each of the main colours (preferably with holes in them and kept in a screw-top jar with some nylon thread)

— a matching test of vision
— a pencil torch (or auriscope/ophthalmoscope)
— pencil and paper
— useful extras are:
— several toy cars, to interest a child without revealing your test kit
— some cake decoration pellets, for a crude vision test and to test pincer grip
— doll-size toys, eg. cup and saucer, hairbrush, shoes
— Ladybird books, for interest and to stimulate conversation
— lift-out puzzles, for the same purpose

SUMMARY OF A BASIC SCREENING SCHEDULE

At 6 – 8 weeks

Skull	— head circumference (on chart)	Hips	— no clunk
	— fontanelles		— full abduction
Eyes	— no cataracts	Feet	— no talipes
	— follows face	Reflexes	— not excessively brisk
Smiles			— fading stepping and Moro reflexes
Hearing	— ask Mother	Anus	
Palate	— intact	Spine	— no lipoma or hair over sacrum
Skin	— any marks		
Heart	— no murmurs		— no abnormal curves
Abdomen	— liver edge only	Tone	— not excessively floppy nor extended
	— no spleen or kidneys		
Genitalia		Posture	— symmetrical limb movements
			— can lift head briefly when prone
		Weight	— in normal range (on chart)
		Length	— ditto (if it can be accurately measured

At 7 – 9 months

Eyes	— no squint	Motor	— sits alone at least briefly
Hearing	— good response to soft high and low-tones each side (see description of test)		— takes weight on feet
			— hips have full abduction
Manipulation	— takes object in either hand and changes hands	Speech	— babbles
		Head circumference and weight	— in normal range (on chart)

At 18 months

Eyes	— no squint	Motor	— walks alone or with minimal support
Hearing	— if still co-operative for a distraction test		— climbs up and down stairs by some method
Manipulation	— piles 3 bricks		— can throw a ball forwards
	— pincer grip of pellet	Speech	— says 6 words with meaning
	— ceased casting one object on floor when second offered		— jabbers to himself
	— ceased mouthing objects		— understands simple commands

Immunisations complete

Height, weight and head circumference charted

At 3 years

Visual acuity —	⎱ see test descriptions	Speech	— using simple sentences well
Hearing —	⎰		— understands use of common objects eg. cup, brush, shoes, etc.
Manipulation	— imitates brick, bridge		— understands quite complex commands eg. "Go upstairs and get Daddy's shoes from the wardrobe".
	— imitates drawing straight lines and circle		
Motor	— can jump		— listens to a short story
	— can stand on one leg (testing each leg)		

Toilet trained by day at least

Height and weight measurements charted
Physical examination if being seen by a doctor

At or just before school entry (4 – 5 years)

Height and weight measurements
   charted
Vision and hearing
Physical examination (if being seen by
   a doctor) of
          — throat and teeth
          — ears
          — heart and chest
          — femoral pulses and
            testes
          — spine
          — reflexes

Manipulation — copies circle, square
                and attempts
                triangle
            — does up most of
                buttons
Motor   — balances on one leg
            — stands on tip-toes
            — easily pedals tricycle
                or bicycle with
                stabilisers
Speech   — clear sentences with
                reasonable
                grammar
            — explains a picture
            — listens to stories or
                TV programme

5

Immunisation

Immunisation is the most obvious preventive medicine that we practise and its effectiveness has made whole generations of the population ignorant of the devastating illnesses that have nearly disappeared. Those of us in our forties can just remember polio as a dread disease but diphtheria had been virtually driven away before we were born. This lack of experience of death and disability from common infectious illnesses tends to make the population, both lay and professional, careless about the importance of immunising every baby. As a nation we cling, probably foolishly, to the civil liberty of keeping this a matter for voluntary parental consent rather than adopting the system used in many countries of making full immunisation a compulsory prerequisite for entering school.

Doctors and nurses are generally concerned with the health needs of individuals, but in the case of immunisation, we also have a responsibility to the community as a whole. For example, when the percentage of children being immunised against whooping cough dropped very low in the late 1970s, an epidemic of the disease occurred which caused death or damage, not necessarily to the children who had not been immunised, but to the youngest members of the community—babies too young to even be eligible for immunisation themselves.

CONSENT FOR IMMUNISATION

This has to be obtained very early in a child's life if he is to start his primary course of immunisation at the correct age of 12 weeks. It sometimes alarms parents to be asked to sign for this series of assaults on their new baby and they must be given sufficient time to allow for informed discussion. The usual problems presented, either at this point or on the day of the first immunisation, are:

1 'I Don't Want Him to Have the Whooping Cough Vaccine'

Firstly, ask why not, because it may be there are members of the family who have epilepsy, or they know someone who is thought to have been brain-damaged by the vaccine. Whether there is a good reason (see next page) for the above statement or not, the very baldness of it should make you aware that the mother feels very strongly about the whole subject. Remember that although you have a duty to do your best for the child by putting the pros and cons as clearly as possible, at the end of the

27

discussion, the final decision belongs to the parents. If you have a flaming row with the mother, not only will you fail to persuade her of the logic of your arguments, but you may also prejudice her against coming to the clinic again. This may seem obvious, but there are some parents who think they know what your attitude will be, and have come determined to fight for what they consider to be right.

2 'I Don't Know if He Should Have the Whooping Cough Injection'

The factors involved are:

(a) No immunisation should be given during an acute febrile illness, including diarrhoea and vomiting, but a runny nose for a few days in an otherwise well baby can be ignored. A child who is nearing the end of a course of antibiotics and has clinically recovered can also safely be immunised.

(b) No immunisation should be given to children being treated for serious illness with cytotoxic drugs and/or steroids, nor to any child with a proven immune deficiency state.

(c) If a severe febrile or neurological reaction occurs after any immunisation, the offending antigen should not be given again. The 'normal' reaction to triple antigen can be a tender red area at the injection site and mild miseries and slight fever for 12 hours. A very swollen arm, persisting high fever and marked irritability is an excessive reaction. (Any such reaction should be notified to the Committee on Safety of Medicines.)

(d) Fits in the neonatal period, cerebral irritation of significant degree or any signs of neurological damage are contra-indications to pertussis immunisation at an early age. If it becomes clear later that the child has no persisting neurological or developmental problems the immunisation can be considered later, preferably with a paediatrician's opinion, up to a maximum of six years of age. This is the most difficult of the contra-indications and examples may be useful. A child who has had a difficult delivery, was jittery for the first 24–48 hours of life or had apnoeic episodes in this time, but no fits, may have no neurological damage but this is difficult to be sure of by the time of the first immunisation. A child who has a known abnormality such as Down's syndrome or spina bifida often remains unimmunised, yet this is really quite illogical. In each case, the wisest course of action is to start the immunising course with diphtheria, tetanus and polio, but once you, the parents and the child's paediatrician are satisfied that there are no neurological abnormalities, a pertussis course should then be started.

(e) Idiopathic epilepsy in first-degree relatives (parents and siblings of the child) are similarly contra-indications to early pertussis immunisation but could be reconsidered later. Febrile convulsions or traumatic epilepsy in a parent are not contra-indications.

Discussion points which may be made to help uncertain parents in their decision are that brain damage from whooping cough itself is more common than from the vaccine; that the majority of doctors, including both of us, have never seen a child who has had a serious reaction to the vaccine, whereas we frequently see children with unpleasant injuries from accidents in their own homes so that, logically, parents should stop agonising over an unlikely risk, when they may be ignoring real ones; that a child with whooping cough is ill and may be very distressing to his parents who feel helpless when he is coughing and vomiting and then wish that they had had him immunised (a tape recording of a child with whooping cough can be very convincing); and lastly, one can blame the media for overdramatising the dangers of the vaccine in the mid-70s which led to the real drama of an epidemic of whooping cough five years later.

Sometimes it is appropriate to make a clear recommendation to uncertain parents that, on balance, in their case, this is what you think best. At other times, it is better to give parents another week to think about their decision, perhaps lending them the latest D.H.S.S. circular to read for themselves.

3 'I Don't Know if He Should Have the Measles Injection'

The factors listed above for pertussis vaccine also apply to measles, except for (c), measles immunity being gained by only one injection of antigen. The fact that it is not given until the child is over a year old makes it easier to assess the importance of (d) and (e) and, in any case, where there is doubt about a child's past or family history, specific immune globulin should be given at the same time as measles vaccine to reduce the possibility of an excessive reaction.

Egg sensitivity used to be a contra-indication to measles immunisation because of the way the vaccine was prepared, but it now only applies if it is of such a degree that the child needs hospitalisation as a result of eating eggs, which is very rare.

One of the biggest problems in maintaining a good rate of uptake of measles immunisation is that the disease itself tends to be looked on as a minor childhood illness which many of us endured without lasting damage. It is necessary then to explain to some parents (and professional colleagues) the unpleasantness of the illness, its epidemic nature and common complications and, for this purpose, a photograph of a measles-covered prostrate child with photophobia may be useful without being unreasonably alarmist.

4 'I Don't Believe in Injections'

This may mean anything from a strong belief that immunisation is basically wrong to a fear of needles. As in (1) above, a calm acceptance of the statement, followed by 'What is it that troubles you about injections?' may open a way to sensible discussion. Sometimes all that is needed is to arrange for a member of the clinic staff to hold the baby instead of the parent for immunisations to be given. In a few cases it is clear that this child is just not going to be immunised but, even then, some parents will agree to a course of oral polio immunisation. It is as well to ask if the parents were themselves immunised, since these strongly held beliefs are often passed on by families, and if not, they may also accept polio immunisation at the same time as their child.

THE IMMUNISATIONS THEMSELVES

The nationally-recommended programme (which changes from time to time) is to give triple vaccine with polio at three months, five months and 10 – 11 months, and measles vaccine at 14 months. There is, at present, some contro- versy between different experts about when to begin immunising premature babies. As these babies are particularly at risk from pertussis, and have few reactions, we suggest that immunisation should be begun at 12 weeks from birth.

If a child's primary course is not completed, it can be restarted at whatever point it ceased as though no interruption had occurred. If the primary course is incomplete by 14 months, measles vaccine can still be given at that age (provided it is at least three weeks after the previous immunisation) and the triple and polio course finished later on. The site of injection should be the anterolateral aspect of the thigh or the upper arm. It is important to inject quite deeply, whether intramuscularly or deep subcutaneously, otherwise an unsightly 'sterile cyst' may be formed in the skin. If this should occur, it can be guaranteed to disappear eventually but it may take months to do so and causes anxiety to the child's family.

At the time of the first or second immunisation, it is a good opportunity to re-check the baby's hips, unless this is a routine part of a developmental screening examination during the middle of the first year of life.

The 'pre-school booster' of diphtheria, tetanus and polio immunisation can be given at any time from 4¼ years onwards and is a good opportunity to see the child before school entry, if a routine examination is not done for this purpose. Giving oral polio at this age is much easier if it is disguised on a sugar lump but that hardly seems a good dental principle. Mixing the polio drops with a single drop of syrup on a spoon may be preferable.

REACTIONS TO IMMUNISATION

It is common for a baby to be slightly fretful and have a tender area at the injection site for about 12 hours after injection and parents should be warned of this. It has already been mentioned that a high temperature or fierce local reaction are reasons for omitting the offending antigen next time and it is likely that this will have been pertussis. Any other reaction—prolonged fever, prolonged screaming, convulsion—are all rare and should be referred for consultant opinion, since diagnosis at that stage is important for medicolegal reasons.

After measles immunisation there is no reaction for six or seven days, then a few children develop a measles-like illness for about 24 hours. It is as well to warn mothers of this possibility so that they know what it is if it does happen.

Anaphylactic shock is exceedingly rare following immunisation. The child may suddenly become very flushed, have difficulty breathing, go floppy and unconscious or he may become suddenly pale, and vomit. The management is

— maintain an airway;

— give adrenaline 1:1,000 by intramuscular slow injection of 0.01 ml/kg body weight, which works out at about 0.1 mls for a one-year-old, followed by a further injection of the same amount in two or three minutes' time if not improved;

— steroids given intravenously, or intramuscularly if necessary, may also help and will certainly not worsen the situation;

— hospitalise the child as soon as possible;

— adrenaline 1:1,000 should always be to hand when immunising and should be regularly checked that it is clear and in date.

RECORDING IMMUNISATIONS

Many district health authorities, family practitioner committees and a number of individual general practices have immunisation records on computer, which makes it easy not only to refer to the immune status of individuals but also to find the percentage uptake within the community, or small sections of it. Whatever the system, it should produce names and addresses of persisting defaulters so that they can be followed-up and their parents encouraged to allow a complete course of immunisation to be given. The recording system should also be able to hold information on the reasons for non-immunisation or incomplete courses so that ways can be found to overcome some of the problems, eg. by setting up a home-visiting immunisation team in areas with no local transport or a particularly poor rate of compliance.

It should be important for all of us to know what antigens have been introduced into our bodies and to what diseases we can expect to have immunity, yet few people show much interest in this once the procedure is over. It is a useful health education aspect for clinic staff to encourage the use of a personal immunisation record card to diminish this indifference and emphasise the health-saving, life-saving purpose of immunisation.

Part II

COMMON PHYSICAL PROBLEMS

6

The Skin

RASHES

Eczema — Atopic Dermatitis

'Has he got eczema?

For no very good reason, some parents get unduly worried by the thought of eczema. In fact, many children have a few patches of dry skin, often on the back in one-year-olds, and behind the knees and at the elbows in 2-4-year-olds. There is usually a family history of eczema or asthma, and some children seem worse in hot weather, while others are worse in the cold. The great majority of these will be so mild that it is nothing more than an occasional inconvenience which has completely disappeared by the age of five. For them we would recommend simple general measures to stop the skin becoming too dry by 'avoiding soap and water' (which usually delights the older ones). After that it is useful to have an ascending list of treatments which can be used as necessary.

Parents seem to find it helpful to realise that there are no once-and-for-all cures but that for much of the time the eczema will cause no trouble, only having occasional flareups in certain weather conditions or when the child is ill. They should know when to use the treatments they have been given, and that if those fail, they can always come to the surgery for something stronger.

Treatments—in ascending order of potency:

1 Bath on alternate days, or less often; no long soaks; no bubble bath, etc.
2 Use soap sparingly and only where needed. 'Simple Soap' may cause less trouble than other soaps (no colour or perfume added).
3 Oilatum Emollient—three capfuls to the bath water (available on prescription) 'keeps the skin moist'.
4 Emulsifying ointment may be used in place of soap, or in the bath water by pouring very hot water over a dollop on a teaspoon (available on prescription).
5 1% hydrocortisone rubbed twice a day into any patch which is red and irritant. Ointment may make more of a mess of the clothes than cream, but is more effective. May be used anywhere, including the face.
6 Potent steroid ointments (e.g. Betnovate) should be used sparingly for short periods on those patches not responding to hydrocortisone, but never on the face.

35

7   In the very few patients who have not responded to the above, we would enquire about precipitating factors (for example, furry pets, washing powders, flowers, dust) and refer the child to a dermatologist, although this seldom seems to be necessary.

Cradle Cap (Seborrhoea Capitis)

Both this and miliaria (see under) are only a problem in the first few months—at about three months of age the skin seems to change and they usually disappear shortly afterwards. There is no mistaking cradle cap for anything else. It starts with a dry scaliness of the scalp and rapidly progresses to the typical thick yellow patches. The old-fashioned remedy is to soften the plaques with olive oil (any vegetable oil will do) and then rub them with a firm brush. One of us used a nailbrush on her children, but although it did not hurt, it was only moderately successful: a more effective remedy is to wash the scalp with a cetrimide shampoo which can be bought as such at the chemist or under certain trade names.

Prickly Heat—Miliaria (Which is Neither Malaria nor Milia)

This is a sweat rash which occurs mainly on the scalp and forehead, where obstruction to the openings of the sweat glands produces many tiny vesicles. The baby looks red and hot and the treatment is quite simply to cool him down. A dusting powder may also be helpful.

A sweat rash sometimes extends into a weeping eczematous dermatitis with maceration of the skin and scaling, particularly round the ears. In these cases, it may be difficult to decide whether this is miliaria or eczema or a combination of both. However, no matter what you call it, and in spite of its unpleasant appearance, it responds excellently within two or three days to 1% hydrocortisone lotion dabbed on with cotton wool three times a day.

Infantile Acne (see colour plate)

Rarely in infants we see a genuine acne on the cheeks. It is usually best left without any specific treatment other than soap and water. However, if severe, it may require antibiotics by mouth.

Septic Spots

Some babies develop pustules on the skin with a slight redness round them. One or two in an otherwise healthy baby can be ignored, but, if there are several, or the baby seems to be unwell and is not feeding properly, it is probably safest to treat him with antibiotics. As the pustules are almost always due to a staphylococcus, cloxacillin or an ampicillin/cloxacillin combination would be the drug of choice.

NAPPY RASHES

Eczematous, Infective (Candida), Irritant (Ammonia) (see colour plates)

There are three causes of nappy rash and a few simple questions, as well as examining the baby, will help to sort them out, although you should remember that two or three causes are often present at one time.

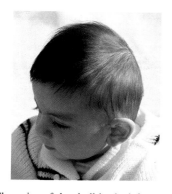

1. Flattening of the skull in the left occipital region. The skull circumference is normal and the child is of normal intelligence. (See p. 40).

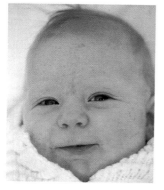

2. Cephalhaematomata. Both parietal bones have a cephalhaematoma. Note that they are clearly limited by the skull sutures. At this stage they are fluctuant but may well calcify when they are as large as this. (See p. 40).

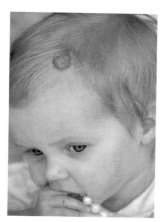

3. Stork Mark. An ill-defined purplish mark between the eyebrows. (See p. 38).

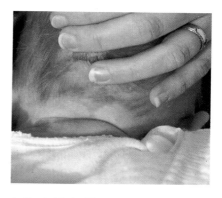

4. Stork Mark. The matching mark to 3 (in the same baby) situated in the hair line at the nape of the neck. Both marks will usually have faded by 4 months.

5. Cavernous Haemangioma (Strawberry mark). Typically raised with a well-defined edge, this one has stopped growing larger and is beginning to fibrose in its centre as the first step to disappearing. (See p. 38).

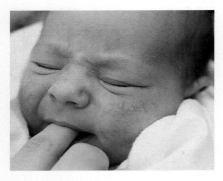

6. Infantile Acne. If purulent and inflamed may need antibiotics by mouth.

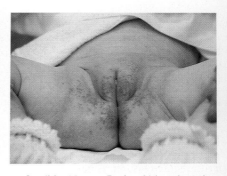

7. Candida Nappy Rash. Although quite mild, this rash shows separate spots some of which are weeping, which is typical of candida. (See p. 37).

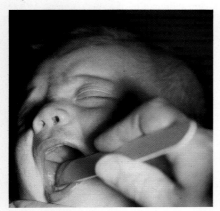

8. Oral Candidiasis. White patches on the buccal mucosa of the same child as in 7. They cannot be wiped off with a spatula and are therefore not milk curds.

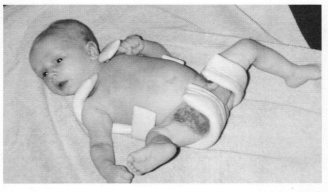

9. Congenital Dislocation of the Hip being treated with a Von Rosen splint. He has developed the unusual complication of a severe nappy rash under the splint of an eczematous type, super-infected by candida. The splint was changed to a Pavlik harness and the rash resolved rapidily. (See p. 54).

'For how long has he had the rash?'

Eczematous rashes are rare before three months, but after that the eczematous child may well have a bit of redness in the nappy area for many months at a time. A sudden onset makes you suspect that there is some aggravating factor, leading you to ask:

'Does the nappy smell strongly of ammonia in the mornings?' and
'Have you changed your washing powder or the way you rinse the nappies?'

The Examination

The bright red rash exactly covering the nappy area is obviously due to an irritant such as ammonia, or a detergent or rinse-aid, and it may be being aggravated by a tight plastic cover to the nappy. Both plastic pants and the modern, tailored disposable nappies can fit so closely that even when a child is 'dry' the skin is kept moist with sweat. Separate bright red spots, some of which are ulcerated, are usually due to *Candida* (thrush): these may be very sore and make the baby cry when wet, or when being washed. If there are patches of dry skin elsewhere on the child then eczema is present.

Discussion and General Treatment

Quite a few young mothers will worry over a slight redness which is very mild to experienced eyes, and really all they need is reassurance and some suggestions about general management.

1 Avoid plastic pants. Plastic ties (Snibs) are a reasonable compromise between letting some air get in to the skin and letting everything else become soaked.
2 Use a simple barrier cream at nappy changes, (zinc & castor oil, Drapolene, etc.)
3 Expose the nappy area for an hour or two each day, if possible. A baby can be left lying on top of a nappy in a warm room, while in summer a toddler can play outside wearing only a top.
4 Rinse out the nappies thoroughly at the end of the wash, if washing them by hand.
5 If possible, try not to leave the baby wet for too long.

Specific Treatments

1 Eczematous rashes will often respond to the above measures, otherwise, 1% hydrocortisone ointment, or as a very last resort, Betnovate ointment, both of them applied about two or three times a day.
2 *Candida* seems to respond well to nystatin, but if it keeps coming back it may also be present in the mouth, the whole alimentary tract and, of course, in the mother. Nystatin drops may be needed for the child (see Oral thrush), and appropriate treatment for the mother.

If both eczema and *Candida* are present, one of us sometimes uses Timodine, and if that does not work, Trimovate. However, this is getting into the realms of blunderbuss therapy, for use by those who cannot make a diagnosis.

3   Ammonia dermatis will usually be obvious to the mother by the strong smell of ammonia present when a wet nappy has been on for some hours. This is caused by the urea in the urine breaking down chemically, and can be stopped very simply by adding a tablespoonful of vinegar to the final rinse when the nappies are washed. The weak acid (acetic acid) in vinegar prevents the chemical breakdown. Soaking nappies in Nappisan or similar agents is also useful in helping to prevent urea breakdown.

BIRTH MARKS

Stork Marks (see colour plates)

'What's this mark on the back of his neck?'

A stork mark is a common, purple-coloured mark which is present at the nape of the neck and between the eyebrows in young babies. The mother can be reassured that it is of no significance and will usually disappear after about three months. The true explanation is uncertain, but may be due to pressure on the foetal skull where it was engaged in the mother's pelvis during the last months of pregnancy. However, the traditional explanation of it being the points at which the stork held the baby when delivering it, is not only picturesque but it is helpful by implying (correctly) that the mark is of no consequence.

Mongolian Blue Spot

This is a dark blue patch present at birth, and usually sited on the lower part of the back or on the thighs. To an outsider it can look like a bruise, but most mothers know what it is and are not concerned by it. It is common in babies of Negro, Asian and Mediterranean races, but there is little point in mentioning this fact, since people from this stock may feel you are being racist, while Caucasians may think you are doubting their pedigree. No treatment is needed and it fades during the first few months.

Strawberry Naevus (Cavernous Haemangioma) (see colour plate)

'He's got this red mark on his chest and it's growing bigger'

A strawberry mark is bright red and raised with a rather rough surface. It can occur at any site, but is most frequently seen on the scalp or trunk. Although it is seldom present at birth, it appears soon afterwards, and can grow rapidly up to the age of about a year. It may also extend underneath the skin to produce a very large swelling.

No treatment is needed, and provided you are sure of the diagnosis, you should resist all pressures to 'do something'. It begins to clear by developing white patches of fibrosis in the middle, and these will slowly spread until the whole mark has disappeared leaving normal skin. This usually occurs in the second year, but may be later, and it almost always seems to have gone by the age of four. A dermatologist's opinion would probably only be called for if a naevus persisted after that age. You should explain to the mother that any attempts at treatment are likely to lead to a scar, although this advice may change if current advances in laser treatment alter the management.

Port-Wine Stain (Capillary Haemangioma)

'Will this mark go?'

A port-wine stain is the same purplish colour as a stork mark, but is brighter and has clear cut edges. It is much the most significant of the skin marks found on babies because it is present for life. Obviously, this is of little importance when the lesion is a small one on some obscure part of the body, but when it is on the face the parents naturally become worried about it.

There is no treatment which can successfully remove a port-wine stain, but if the parents are distressed by it, they may be able to accept the inevitable more easily with a second opinion. They may also find it helpful to realise that they are the people who can most help their child, by taking a positive attitude and not letting people's reactions affect him. Finally, masking creams can be prescribed which match the natural skin colour of the child.

7

Head and Neck

THE SKULL

Fontanelle (Soft Spot)

'Will it hurt him if I wash his soft spot?'

Mothers often seem to think that the brain lies immediately under the skin at the fontanelle. You can mention that not only are there scalp muscles under the skin, but that the skull bones are joined by a tough membrane. Unless they start hammering nails through it, they would probably have a hard job to make any impression on the brain. It may also forestall worries if you point out that the fontanelle varies greatly in size from baby to baby and in the speed at which it is turned into bone, so that while it has usually almost closed by the first birthday, it is quite normal to take several months longer.

Cephalhaematoma (see colour plate)

'What's this lump on his head?'

Bumps and bruises on the scalp from a traumatic delivery mostly disappear within the first week after birth. A cephalhaematoma on the other hand is a subperiosteal haematoma over one of the skull bones, and is therefore limited to the area of that bone by the periosteum (which is the reason why it is poorly reabsorbed). It is often seen at the eight-week check and may calcify. Apart from the unusual shape, this does not matter in the least: as the skull grows and the cranium is remodelled, the lump is absorbed so that it will have disappeared completely by the age of one year. The only thing the parents need to do is to keep it covered to protect themselves from rude comments ('Oh dear, did the little fellow fall on his head?').

Flattening (see colour plate)

'Why is his head flat on this side?'
'Why is his head lopsided?'

A baby will naturally tend to turn his head towards the light, so if he always lies with the light on one side the occiput becomes flattened on that side. The simple remedy is to turn the baby round so that his head lies at the other end of the cot, and the light is therefore on his other side. In fact a bit of uneveness is usual at about three months, and this tends to even up by about eight months when the baby is sitting for much of the day.

40

Funnily-Shaped Heads.

It is not uncommon to see babies with a head that is long and thin, or fat at the back, and the former is particularly common in premature babies. These shapes are of no significance in themselves, and you will frequently only need to take one look at the parents to see where it comes from. The crucial factor is whether the child has a normal head circumference compared with its weight, and whether this is increasing at a normal rate. The birth measurement of the head should be available at child health clinics as a baseline, and it is always possible to bring the child back in a week to recheck it. However, if there is any doubt, the child should be referred either to a neurosurgeon or a paediatrician without delay, since the consequences of untreated hydrocephalus are so serious.

FACE AND MOUTH

Cleft Palate

In the majority of cases a cleft palate will be picked up shortly after birth and referred to a plastic surgeon before the child ever reaches a child health clinic. However, it is always worth getting a look at the palate during the eight-week check, and occasionally you will find a bifid uvula, or minor degree of cleft in the soft palate. The plastic surgeons like to see anything that involves the palate, and even the clearly bifid uvula, since these may be associated with abnormal musculature to the palate. There is nothing to be gained from delaying referral.

On discussing a cleft palate with the mother you will be able to say that repair is usually carried out before six months with excellent results. In some children with a very wide cleft, an orthodontic plate may be needed first, which helps feeding and narrows the cleft. Some affected babies find it difficult to suck and need spoon feeding, but this will have been discovered in hospital and the mother should merely need support from the clinic staff over the first few months.

Speech Problems with Cleft Palates

The typical 'nasal escape' type of speech seems now to be less common, which is probably due to more complete and effective repairs. However, most children will benefit from speech therapy, and here again the speech therapists like to get to work with the child and the parents at an early age. Usually, there is very close cooperation between plastic surgeons and the speech therapy department, but the clinic doctor should just make sure that the latter know about the child by the time he is three.

Hare Lip

A hare lip is a horrific deformity to a mother longing for a perfect baby. In actual fact, all hare lips are repaired within the first three months with amazingly good results. The majority of hare lips are nowadays completely corrected at the first operation, but some children may be left with flattening of the nose which is usually corrected at about four years of age before they start school.

Here again, referral will have taken place before the child is seen at the clinic, and the role of the clinic staff lies in supporting the mother. It is usually inappropriate for the baby to be brought up to a public clinic before he has had surgery, as this will cause the mother acute embarrassment and unhappiness. However, it is most important that he is visited regularly by the health visitor and doctor, who can ensure that the feeding is satisfactory and that plans for surgery are progressing. In particular, the parents are encouraged if they can see photographs and booklets explaining what is done and when. Surgery normally requires about a week's stay in hospital.

Bat Ears

Quite a lot of children have ears that stick out a bit. In a true bat ear, the pinna has lost the normal folds in its cartilage so that it sticks straight out. This may not bother the child too much and plastic surgeons like to take the child's own feelings into account when deciding upon surgery. For this reason there is very little point in referring children before the age of six. However, the point should also be made to the child and his parents that this is a common problem with a low priority, so there is often a long wait before surgery is actually performed.

Teething

'Should he have some teeth by now?'

Most babies produce their first teeth at six to eight months, but it is normal for this to happen at any time from birth until after the first birthday. In fact, occasionally newborn babies have little deciduous teeth which drop out in the first few weeks. Whatever happens, the age at which the teeth appear is unimportant and cannot be altered.

'He's got this rash and a temperature, but he's teething!'

So many illnesses are ascribed to teething that we find ourselves constantly repeating the motto 'Teething never made any child ill'. Some babies are fractious when teething, and most are certainly keen to gnaw objects as well as dribbling a lot, but you must start looking for causes of infection if a mother says that her baby has a temperature. It is also unusual for children to go off their food when teething. Indeed, this is perhaps the most significant of all signs that a child has something more than a trivial illness.

For treatment, we would usually recommend that the child is given things to chew, such as teething rings and toast. If he seems very irritable and will not settle at night, the occasional dose of paracetamol syrup may then be helpful, but if this is needed much, you must be looking for something more than teething. We have not found patent preparations which can be rubbed on gums to be of much use.

Oral Thrush—Candidiasis (see colour plate)

Infection in the mouth with candida is common in babies during the first three months. It may indicate that the whole gut is infected and be associated with a candida nappy rash, or it may be totally asymptomatic. It appears as white curds, usually situated on the buccal mucosa, although it can also be on the tongue. To differentiate it from milk curds, you should gently scrape it with a spatula when it will be found to adhere to the mucosa or bleed if it is scraped off, unlike normal milk curds. It usually responds well to a one week course of nystatin drops given 3 times a day after feeds (so that they are not washed away by the feeds). Resistant infections are best ignored if they are asymptomatic, or otherwise they may be treated with amphotericin drops.

Epstein's Pearls

Mothers sometimes notice white shiny pearly lumps on the hard palate in young babies. These are normally in the midline and are called Epstein's Pearls. They are harmless, cause no problems and disappear naturally.

EYE CONDITIONS

Squints—Lazy Eye (Strabismus)

'Do you think he is squinting?'

The History Before you check any child for a squint it is worth making sure that you are talking about the same thing as the parents (some people mean screwing the eyes up when they talk about squinting). It is then helpful to know when the squint occurs and how often. In the majority of children who develop one, it is first noticed between the ages of six and 18 months, and is usually seen intermittently at first, particularly when the child is tired or ill. In these cases there is frequently a strong family history of squints and, conversely, if such a family history exists, you need then to be particularly on the lookout in siblings. Before the age of four months, control of the eye movements is rather haphazard, and a baby tends not to fixate on anything for more than a second or two at a time. However, at this early age an inability to fix at all, or a clear cut squint, can both be pointers to more serious eye conditions such as blindness, cataracts or retinoblastoma.

Testing for a Squint To check for a squint, it is best to have the child sitting on the parent's lap, level with you and with the light shining onto the child from behind you. A manifest squint is obvious and can be confirmed by the light reflex (reflection of the light) being at a different point on each of the child's eyes.

symmetrical (normal)   asymmetrical

Fig 7.1 Test for squint—light reflex

It may also show up more clearly on lateral gaze if you move a bright object from side to side in front of him. In a child who is just beginning to develop a squint, there may be nothing to see, but a latent squint can be detected by the cover test. For this you simply cover one eye with your hand, get the child to look at an object with the other eye and then remove your hand. If there is a latent squint present, the covered eye will not be looking at the object, and after removing the cover, it will either remain looking in the wrong direction or you will see it move into the correct position.

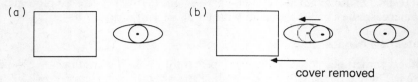

Fig 7.2 Test for squint—cover test. A: Left eye looking at object, right eye covered; B: On removal of cover, left eye remains looking at object—right eye may remain looking inwards (or outwards) or may also move to fix on object

Many of us have great difficulty in deciding whether or not a child has a squint when he also has a very wide bridge to his nose, (a broad epicanthus). It sometimes helps to get him to follow an object like a pen: as you bring it straight towards his nose and then away again, you should see the eyes converge equally and then diverge.

Management Squints should be referred promptly because of the need to exclude underlying conditions, and to begin treatment as early as possible. Even when you cannot detect a squint, you should still ask for a second opinion if the mother is pretty certain that it is present at times. You can tell the mother that if one is confirmed, early treatment gets excellent results and is aimed at preventing a lazy eye (amblyopia), that is, where the vision is lost in one eye because it has not been used. The usual line of treatment starts with patching of the good eye, followed, if necessary, by surgery to the eye muscles, and glasses. Young children withstand such intrusions on their liberty with surprisingly little fuss provided the parents are quietly insistent.

Sticky Eyes

Babies frequently get watering of one or both eyes with crusting on the eyelids. This is of no great significance, and is treated by bathing the eyes with warm water on cotton wool. If the discharge persists or becomes obviously purulent, or the conjunctiva becomes red, a course of antibiotic eye drops should then be given. Chloramphenicol is the drug of choice and should be used about every two hours because the drops tend to wash away. They are usually effective within three days, and if there is no improvement in that time the parent should bring him back. A persistent discharge from both eyes which is very purulent, can be caused by infection in the nose and postnasal space, and may be due to pneumoccoci. In this case antibiotics by mouth will be more effective.

Blocked Tear Ducts

'He's got a sticky eye again'
  When this occurs for the third time in the first three months, the mother may feel that you are not treating the condition correctly, or that she is once

again demonstrating her incompetence by failing to look after her baby properly. Of course, neither is true. Blocked tear ducts are common in babies and often seem to persist until about nine months, when the majority of them clear spontaneously. The affected eye will tend to water, particularly in the cold wind, and have crusts along the eyelashes. It will also be more liable to infection. If the mother understands this, she is usually quite happy to bathe the eye more frequently and only bring the baby back to the doctor if it becomes frankly purulent. Those children who are still having problems at nine months can be referred to an eye department where the usual treatment is to probe the ducts with a bristle under anaesthetic.

NECK

'What's this lump in his neck?'

Cervical Glands

Most children have a bout of tonsillitis at some time before the age of five, and many of them will develop large cervical glands. Parents can usually accept those at the common site below the angle of the jaw, but tend to become worried when lumps appear at the occiput or lying on top of the sternomastoids. Underlying their anxiety is the fear that it is 'cancer' or 'leukaemia' and, of course, in the experience of most GPs this fear will prove correct two or three times during their career.

If the child is eating normally and looks healthy on examination of the nose and throat, you can reassure the mother that the glands must have become enlarged to fight a recent infection, which is, after all, their job. Review the child in a couple of weeks or ask the mother to bring him back if they get larger rather than smaller.

If the child is ill, you will obviously treat him, and if he looks pale it may be worth taking swabs and a blood count. Although you are unlikely to find leukaemia, a simple iron deficiency anaemia is not uncommon, and these children are often a bit 'run-down', being generally miserable and developing frequent infections. On the other hand, when there is bruising, pallor and large glands, you should be much more suspicious and consider immediate referral.

Sternomastoid Tumours—Wry Neck (Torticollis)

A sternomastoid tumour, causing torticollis, is present at birth or soon after. If the baby's head is extended, the 'tumour' is easily seen and the degree of trouble it is causing can be gauged by the amount the head is rotated away from the side of the tumour. Once the parents appreciate that it is merely caused by a 'knotting-up' of the sternomastoid muscle, they find no difficulty in gently stretching it every day by turning the head in the opposite direction. The few children that are not cured by this manoeuvre should be referred between six months of age and one year, because the tumour occasionally needs surgical release.

8

The Body

THE CHEST

Depressed Sternum—Funnel Chest (Pectus Excavatum)

A funnel chest does not seem to alarm parents much, and nor should it. One sometimes sees such a marked depression that it looks as though the sternum must be almost touching the vertebrae. However, this does not impair the child's health in any way, and although the heart is displaced to the left, lung function remains normal. The depression slowly becomes less deep in the years before puberty.

Breast Swelling

Most babies (male and female) have some enlargement of the breast tissue after birth due to the effect of the mother's hormones. In some, a small amount of milky fluid is even secreted, but if the breasts are left alone this settles, although swelling of the nipple may persist for up to about three months.

THE HEART

Heart murmurs in young children are common, although more frequently heard after six months than at the eight-week check. Inevitably, when you hear a murmur you will have to spend longer listening with a stethoscope than usual, and even if she says nothing the mother may be thinking 'Is there something wrong?'. So what, if anything, do you say and do?

Firstly, you have to make some sort of diagnosis to answer for yourself whether or not it is a significant lesion. You are not helped by the fact that while innocent murmurs abound, many cardiac lesions in the first year do not have a murmur or have not developed the murmur that is typically associated with them later on.

Examining the Heart When an Abnormality is Suspected

1   Appearance: Check that the child looks healthy and is not pale or cyanosed and weigh him (significant lesions often cause a poor weight gain).
2   Listen in all areas for a murmur to check its timing, to detect where it can be heard and where it is loudest (particularly the apex, the left sternal border, the pulmonary area and the back). Some murmurs are heard best with a diaphragm and others with a bell; some may be confused by the breath sounds.

46

3 Listen to the second sound over the upper sternum to try and detect whether there is a loud P_2 (raised pulmonary artery pressure) and whether there is a normal split between the aortic and pulmonary second sounds.

4 Feel the chest with the flat of your hand to detect a thrill (usually only present with the louder murmurs), or right ventricular hypertrophy felt over the sternum, or a forceful apex beat indicating left ventricular hypertrophy. NB Right ventricular hypertrophy is common in congenital heart disease.

5 Check the femoral pulses, that they are present and coincide with the pulse at the wrist. In small children and babies it may be easier to detect pulses in the foot.

The typically innocent murmur is an ejection systolic murmur heard loudest at the lower left sternal border, with a 'vibratory' or 'twanging' quality. It does not radiate to other areas and there is a normal pulmonary second sound.

A venous hum is also of no significance. It is usually heard just below the clavicles and is abolished by lying the child slightly head down.

Some Findings Which are Usually Abnormal

Murmurs radiating to the back or the neck.
An ejection click (which is a high-pitched sound, heard after the first heart sound and before the murmur).
A second heart sound which is loud, single, or widely split and does not change with respiration.
A diastolic murmur.
A pan-systolic murmur which obliterates the second heart sound.
A palpable thrill or ventricular hypertrophy.

In the end you should refer children with any of the above, and also any child who is

— unwell or failing to make an average weight gain,
— tachypnoeic, sweaty, or breathless with feeds,
— cyanosed (but even babies with Fallot's may be pink up to one year).

Having decided to refer the child, you can do two things to help to lessen the parents' anxiety. You can do your best to make sure the child gets an out-patient appointment in a reasonably short time, (but you must beware of this being taken to indicate that you think there is something which needs urgent treatment). Secondly, you can reassure the parents that the majority of patients you refer are in fact found to have no significant lesion, because those with serious lesions will almost always have developed symptoms at an earlier age, so they will have already been seen and started on treatment. It is very rare for a major cardiac abnormality to be found in a child health clinic.

Wait and See

A far larger number of children with heart murmurs will not need referral, so what do you say? Many of us find ourselves following Illingworth's advice and saying nothing on the first occasion, provided the mother seems unworried and the child is well. You must make a note in the records and also note that you have not told the mother. Usually you are due to see the child again within six months, when you can decide whether the murmur has altered in that time.

If the murmur remains unchanged, or is louder, you should then tell the parents because it is possible that someone else may notice it at a time when the child is ill, and cause much greater alarm, but you can try to put the whole matter into its true perspective by mentioning three things.

1   The murmur has been there for some months and the child has developed normally in that time.
2   These murmurs are called 'innocent' because that is what they are. It is thought that they are caused by turbulence in the blood flow, possibly because the vessels in a child are narrow and the bends in the great vessels are sharper. However, there is no structural abnormality present.
3   Because they are caused by turbulent flow, the murmurs will vary with changes in the heart rate, so they may either get louder or disappear when the child is exercising or unwell.

If the mother notices you taking a long time examining the heart on any occasion, you will have to discuss the whole matter. Some mothers will say, 'Oh, I've known about that for ages. My doctor mentioned it when we saw him a little while ago'. Others will become inappropriately worried. If the above explanation does not settle them, repeated reassurances merely reinforce the idea that you are hiding the bad news from them. It is better to ask a mother in this state to come back again in a short time with her husband so that you can explain it to him also. If the anxiety still remains, then the time has come for a consultant opinion even though it is not warranted on medical grounds.

Lastly, normal hearts should be treated normally. Innocent murmurs do not warrant any special treatment, nor do they cause recurrent colds, tonsillitis, or any other of the 'thousand natural shocks that flesh is heir to'.

THE ABDOMEN

Umbilical Hernia

'His tummy button sticks out'

About one child in 10 has a small umbilical hernia by the time of the eight-week check. In many of them this will grow more prominent and larger over the next few months, before disappearing spontaneously sometime in the first five years. Although the bulge may be the size of an adult finger the actual defect in the abdominal wall is usually small, and it only needs to grow slightly narrower to prevent the bowel coming through. The old fashioned remedy was to tape a penny over the umbilicus or apply a binder. Not only is this unnecessary, but it is positively dangerous because it can trap the hernia while it is out and lead to bowel necrosis. Unlike inguinal herniae, there is not a risk of obstruction, so there is no need for surgical closure on these grounds. Umbilical herniae are even more common in Negro children where they tend to be larger, and associated with divarication of the recti. However, it still applies that the great majority will close spontaneously and you need only refer those children who still have one at five years. On the other hand, para-umbilical herniae do not close on their own.

Umbilical Granuloma

When the umbilical cord separates, an area of granulation tissue is often left which may grow rapidly rather than epithelialising as it should. The resultant granuloma looks like a small red cherry protruding through the umbilicus.

It is very simple to treat by tying a piece of thread moderately tightly round its base. Although this procedure is painless the baby usually objects to being messed around, so it is helpful to have someone holding him to prevent him from bringing his knees up. If you can find a nurse to be your helper so much the better, because mothers tend to be squeamish about touching the umbilicus.

You may also touch the granuloma with a silver nitrate stick, which helps to dry it up and stop any oozing of blood that may occur. In most cases this is all that is required, and it drops off in about four days. Sometimes a second ligature is needed, a bit tighter than the first.

Inguinal Hernia

'He seems to get a bulge in his groin at times when he is crying'

Occasionally, you will be brought a baby of the two to four-month age group who has an obvious bulge in the inguinal region on one side (sometimes both). More commonly, there will be nothing to see even when the child cries, but the history alone should give you the diagnosis. Most of these will be boys and it is important to know whether the testes were normal and in the scrotum when the lump appeared.

On examination, you may be lucky enough to see the hernia, in which case you should mention that in your referral letter because it may well refuse to make an appearance for the surgeon. If it is not present you may be able to feel thickening of the cord as it passes over the pubis, and sometimes there is an associated hydrocoele. You should look out for the very mobile testis which can sometimes travel from the scrotum high into the superficial inguinal pouch and therefore be misleading.

All inguinal herniae, or suspected herniae, should be referred promptly for a surgical opinion. It is amazing how many of these obstruct in the time between being first noticed and receiving surgery.

Hydrocoele

A hydrocoele is a scrotal swelling full of clear fluid. It is situated in front of the testis, so that a large one may make it impossible to feel the testis. Both hydrocoeles and indirect inguinal herniae are caused by a patent processus vaginalis connecting the tunica vaginalis with the abdominal cavity and they can occur together or occasionally one may develop from the other.

Provided there is no evidence of a hernia, a small hydrocoele can be left alone if it is first seen at the eight-week check or earlier. The majority will disappear spontaneously. However, large or recurrent hydrocoeles should be referred after three months of age.

MALE GENITALIA

Undescended Testicle

'Does it mean he won't be able to have children?'

The easiest time to detect an undescended testicle is during the first few months, when the baby is usually warm and the cremaster muscle is not so active in drawing the testicle up to the neck of the scrotum. Trying to determine whether both testes are descended in five-year-old boys who have been stripped to their underpants while waiting for a school medical can be merely a form of gambling. ('Now you see it; now you don't!'). With proper records from birth, warm hands, and a warm child, the sporting element can be eliminated. It is often easier to detect the testes if the boy is asked to squat in the 'frog position' or to lie down with his thighs flexed.

Surgeons seem to vary about the age at which they like to perform an orchidopexy, but children should be referred at any age when testes cannot be identified in the scrotum and by the age of six, if possible. It is important to impress on the parents that an undescended testicle is likely to function normally if it can be brought into the scrotum. It is therefore up to them to ensure that he receives treatment in good time.

Testicular Torsion

A testicle may suffer from torsion either by rotating within the tunica vaginalis or by the whole cord twisting. In both cases this cuts off the blood supply which runs in the cord, and becomes a surgical emergency. Any child with a painful or swollen testicle should be assumed to have testicular torsion and be referred straight to hospital (it should also be remembered that the pain is sometimes referred to the RIF). Boys who have had an undescended testicle on one side, have a greater risk of this happening on the other side as well.

The Penis

Come back, Freud; all is forgiven!
'Is his Willy too small?'
'Should we pull the foreskin back?'
'Is the little hole too small?'
'Does he need circumcision?'
'Should it have this bend in it?'
'Is it all right for him to keep playing with it?'

Sex being the powerful force that it is, it is hardly surprising that such a disproportionately large number of queries should be raised about so small an organ. Some mothers, in particular, seem obsessed with their son's future ability to satisfy the fair sex, while the medical profession goes through cycles of advising parents in different directions. When you add religious practices to these, you realise that it is the only subject which manages to encompass the prejudices of sex, religion, race and tradition.

Circumcision

Luckily, the question of circumcision on religious grounds is not usually brought to a child health clinic, and in any case it is not allowable under the NHS. For those parents who ask about it on grounds of hygiene and come with an open mind, we recommend circumcision only where necessary. In other words, the foreskin has a role in protecting the glans, and should normally be left alone. Children may be considered for circumcision either because they have had two bouts of balanitis, or because they have a pinhole meatus, after the age of three, which is obstructing urine flow, and this is demonstrated by ballooning of the foreskin on passing water.

The non-retractile foreskin is a subject which has worried parents and doctors over the ages. It must be stressed that it is normal to be unable to retract the foreskin up to the age of three years but after that age, in the great majority of boys, it will be fully retractile, and in the rest the few remaining adhesions can be gently freed with a probe and some local anaesthetic jelly.

When circumcision is requested on religious grounds, it is pointless forcefully to try to dissuade the parents. However, you may point out that every year there are a few deaths in Britain, and a number of repair operations, caused by inexpert attempts at circumcision. Having stated the facts, we think you should then refer them privately to a competent surgeon, rather than see them go to someone less competent.

An absolute contra-indication to circumcision arises when the child has hypospadias of any degree. In these children the extra skin may well be needed at a later stage for the repair operation. If circumcision is still insisted on for religious reasons, the performer can usually be persuaded to only make a ritual nick in the foreskin.

Size

The size of the penis varies enormously, and it may appear particularly small in the chubby child because of the pubic fat. This couldn't matter less. By the time puberty has been reached, it will have enlarged considerably, and be more than equal to the demands made on it. True micropenis is very uncommon but if it occurs you should also bear in mind adrenogenital syndromes.

'Nasty Habits'

It is very common for small boys (and girls) to play with themselves from a few months old. This is perfectly normal and can be ignored, since it does not lead to any problems. If it continues rather blatantly after the age of four just mention to the child that older children and adults do not do so in public. This comment may have more effect coming from the doctor than the parents.

Congenital Abnormalities (Hypospadias)

Glandular or primary hypospadias occurs not infrequently where the foreskin is incomplete on the underside and the urinary meatus is also on the underside of the glans. In practice, little needs to be done, unless there is also some degree of chordee (tightening along the underside of the penis so that it cannot come up to a straight erection). However, you still may wish to refer this at an early stage to a plastic surgeon for his opinion.

In more severe degrees of hypospadias the meatus is situated further down the shaft of the penis or at its base. This will usually have been noted before the child is brought to a clinic, but if it has not been already referred to a plastic surgeon, this should be done.

You can reassure the parents that in these days all degrees of hypospadias are correctable surgically to produce a functioning result, but that on no account must they let their child be circumcised (see above).

FEMALE GENITALIA

A minor degree of fusion of the labia minora in baby girls is common: it often passes unnoticed by the parents and can be left alone. Where it is more marked, the labia can be gently separated with a probe and local anaesthetic cream. The two surfaces should be prevented from fusing again with vaseline, and by separation at least twice a day for two weeks.

After birth, the clitoris is relatively enlarged because of the effect of maternal hormones. Sometimes it is so enlarged that you may consider hermaphoditism, but in practice these all seem to have regressed to more normal proportions by the time of the eight-week check.

Another harmless effect of maternal hormones, or at least of their withdrawal, can be seen in newborn girls who have a vaginal discharge during the first week of life. This is usually creamy, but may be bloodstained within the first month. It is of no significance.

9

Skeletal

INTRODUCTION

Orthopaedic problems are frequently brought to child health clinics, and are usually minor variations of the normal which need no treatment and which become less obvious with time and growth. However, they also include some extremely important conditions which will need the correct treatment if the child is not to be left with a lifelong deformity. The clinic doctor must be able to differentiate these two groups accurately, to avoid either a deluge of pointless referrals or missing treatable conditions.

Many generalised diseases of childhood, especially those of the nervous system, muscles and joints, produce orthopaedic problems. These are best dealt with in a combined clinic of paediatrician and orthopaedic surgeon, but in the absence of such a clinic, the child health doctor or health visitor may usefully liaise between the child's family, his GP and the paediatric and orthopaedic departments. This can certainly help the family to know that the child is seen as a whole and not in anatomical segments and it may well reduce the number of outpatient attendances needed.

THE BACK

Hair, Lumps and Pits on the Back

Many babies have a growth of fine hair spreading over the lower part of the back, and extending up the spine and onto the buttocks. This is commoner in babies from Mediterranean and Indian stock than it is in Northern Europeans, and is of no significance. On the other hand, a distinct tuft of hair at the base of the spine may be an indication of an underlying spina bifida and associated neurological impairment. It should be referred, and a close eye kept on the child's further development. Problems with bladder control and lesser degrees of weakness in the leg muscles may be difficult to detect before the age of two. A low hairline associated with a short neck may be an indication of a Klippel-Feil deformity.

A fatty lump or lipoma over the spine may signify an abnormality of the underlying spine and spinal cord. Although seen most often in the lumbar region, it can occur at other levels, notably over the lower cervical spine. As with hairy tufts, neurological lesions are more likely to be severe when the abnormality is at the L3 level or above, but all the clearly defined ones should be referred.

53

A pit at the upper end of the natal cleft may involve the spinal cord. A dimple is frequently seen at this point, but if the skin is intact nothing more needs to be done. Where the bottom of a pit cannot be seen, it may be continuous with the spinal cord and lead to meningitis, so it must be investigated further.

How far you should take action over what is probably a minor variation from normal in any of these conditions will depend on the lesion and on the services available to you. You can hardly justify causing the parents some years of anxiety if you think there is nothing that needs to be done. In these circumstances we would make sure a baby is moving his legs properly (Moro and Stepping reflexes) and leave it at that, without mentioning anything to the parents, but making sure he is followed in the clinic. If the parents mention the lesion, or there is the least doubt in your mind, the baby should then be referred. Where there is a neurosurgeon who specialises in these problems the choice is easy, but otherwise it may be appropriate to ask a paediatrician or an orthopaedic surgeon to see him. It may often be useful to ask for X-rays of the spine while waiting for the appointment, but these are not enough on their own for you to reassure the parents without a consultant opinion as well.

THE HIPS

Congenitally Dislocated Hips

Although a clicking hip is common in the newborn, one very rarely picks up a dislocated hip in a clinic. This may reflect the quality of the doctors examining newborn babies, but it has the drawback that clinic doctors do not often get the chance to actually feel a hip which dislocates because most will already be in splints by the time of the eight-week check.

Examination for CDH

A At 6-8 Weeks

The hips are best checked by a combination of Barlow's and Ortolani's tests. The baby lies on his back and the thighs are flexed to a right angle with the knees together. Slight downward pressure on the knees will ensure that the hip will have dislocated backwards if that is possible. You then fully abduct the thighs with the tips of your fingers over his greater trochanter. If either hip has dislocated it will slot back into the acetabulum with a clunk that you can feel as you abduct the thighs.

In testing the hips you should beware of clicks from the knee joints. It is also important to have the baby lying reasonably quietly, so if he is screaming for a feed, it is better to let him be fed and test again later.

B At 8 Months

It is strongly recommended that the hips are rechecked at about this age. There is now good evidence that a number of dislocated hips do not present until after the first few months, and these are the ones most in need of treatment. By eight months they are more difficult to check because the children are bigger and

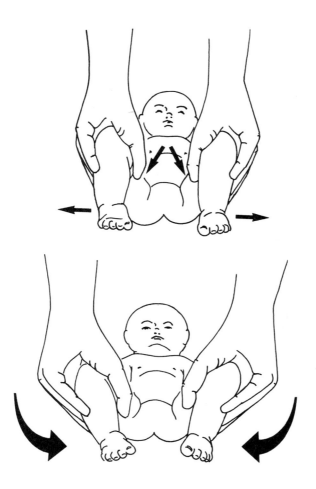

Fig 9.1   Testing for dislocated hips at 6 – 8 weeks

tend to have chubby thighs. However, the absolutely fundamental test is still to abduct the thighs while they are flexed 90° at the hip joint. This should be possible in both legs to a minimum of 60°. You may also like to test for full range of hip movements by seeing if he can suck his toes with each leg in turn while the other leg is kept straight. Other helpful signs of dislocation are, shortening of one leg, asymmetrical creases on the buttocks, and the knees being at different levels when the hips are flexed with the baby lying on his back.

X-rays of the hips can be useful after six months of age, but are notoriously difficult to interpret before then.

For foetal alignment of the hips, see under next section.

THE LEGS

General Examination of the Legs and Feet

'His Foot Turns In!'

This must be the commonest query that mothers raise spontaneously at child health clinics, for the good reason that there is an obvious deformity. You can just hear the grandparents saying 'You must get him seen by the specialist or he'll never walk properly'. The fact is, of course, that most of these conditions are entirely benign and disappear as the child gets older, but for all of them there is a point at which the degree of deformity becomes abnormal and referral is needed.

The basic principles of orthopaedic examination of any child must not be forgotten simply because one is presented in clinic with an apparently healthy child.

Basic Actions at Each Examination:

- look at both sides of the body, not just the affected one
- look at the joints above and below the affected site and test movement
- measure limb length, muscle bulk, etc., as appropriate
- examine the nervous system as well as the bones and joints
- watch the gait and child's ability to get up from lying to standing
- look for any symptom or signs of systemic illness

NB Hot, painful swellings of bones are fractures or osteomyelitis until proved otherwise.

The Examination Technique

Usually the child is just starting to walk, and if you see him walking round holding his mother's hand, he will clearly be tending to turn one foot inwards. Once you have established that you and his mother are talking about the same thing; examine the child on the mother's knee with trousers, tights, shoes and socks off. If you hold the legs out straight together, you will be able to see if the knees point forward in the same direction as the foot when the latter is in the neutral position, i e. not dorsiflexed or extended. Then test the full range of movements of all the joints: beginning with the hips, flex each one and extend it and then with the knee flexed, rotate the hip internally and externally. The mother will usually be amazed to see her child lying quite happily while the leg is rotated through almost 180° so that the lower leg sticks out sideways one minute and is then turned round to point medially the next.

The knees will usually flex and extend normally, and you can then look at the foot and ankle. With the foot held in the neutral position there will be a minor degree of curvature along the inner side, but the line of the forefoot should be straight forward. Check the range of movements at the ankle joint to confirm that dorsiflexion is possible through at least 30°. Extension (plantar flexion) is almost always possible through a good 60°, and the foot can usually be everted and inverted about 30° beyond the neutral, which gives a good indication of suppleness.

The Explanation for Variations from Normal

In most cases the mother will have seen you obtain a wide range of movements at all the joints and you hardly need to say anything else. You can point out that one only has to look at the feet of people walking down the street to see the wide variation between people who walk normally. Secondly, you can make the point that a child's ligaments are very soft and that as he grows they will tend to firm up and the bones to straighten as they respond to the load put on them.

Specific Conditions of the Legs

Knock Knees and Bow Legs

In many toddlers the legs seem to bend either in or out but knock knees and bow legs are physiological in young children.

Early walkers tend to be bandy-legged, while fat girls tend to get knock knees, but neither of these matter, provided the degree of deformity is not too great and there is no underlying pathology.

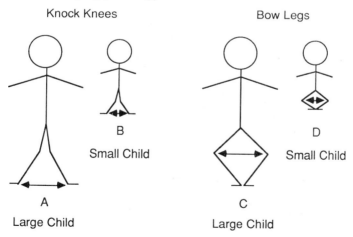

Knock Knees   Bow Legs

B

Small Child

A

Large Child

D

Small Child

C

Large Child

ABCD should all be less than 2.5 in. (6cm)

Fig 9.2   Acceptable normal limits for bow legs and knock knees

To assess their significance you should sit or lie the child down with the legs out straight, and remember the magic figure of 2½" (6cm). In knock knees, with the inside of the knees just touching, the medial malleoli should not be wider than 2½″ apart, and vice versa in bow legs. If the gap is wider, the child should be referred whatever his age or size. This is because the gap should become proportionately smaller as the child gets larger.

With bow legs, the possibility of rickets must be born in mind, particularly with Asian children. In these cases the child will be smaller than average and there may be epiphyseal swelling at the knees and wrists. You may even see the 'rickety rosary' of swellings at the costochondral junctions forming a ring round the sternum, and the child usually appears miserable.

Any asymmetrical knee deformity should also be referred since it suggests some form of pathology of the bones or epiphyses.

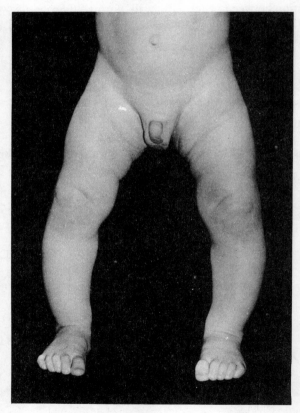

Fig 9.3   Physiological bow legs in a toddler

Foetal Alignment of the Hips—persistent femoral anteversion

Here the whole leg appears to be turned inwards, so that when the child is sitting with his legs straight out in front of him, the knee caps appear to 'squint' inwards. On examining the hips you will find that a large amount of

nternal rotation is possible but only limited external rotation. You can confirm
his by lying the child on his tummy, flexing the knee at 90° and rotating the
eg internally and externally. Referral is only needed if external rotation is less
han 5°, otherwise you can reassure the mother that it will continue to improve
pontaneously up to the age of eight.

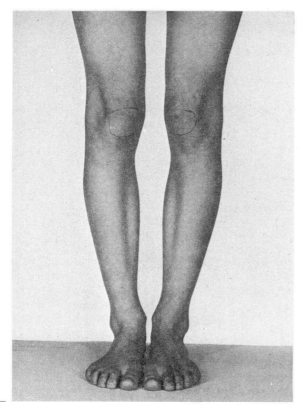

Fig 9.4   Persistent femoral anteversion—note the 'squinting' kneecaps

ibial Torsion

Iere there is a twist along the length of the lower leg so that the foot points in-
vards or outwards when the knee is facing forwards. To confirm the diagnosis
ou should examine the child with the knee flexed and turn the foot in and out
to find the average degree of rotation of the tibia.

Improvement occurs naturally and you only need to refer children whose average
i-toeing is 45° or more, or who are extremely clumsy. Treatment with appliances
i useless and the only effective correction is by surgery, to divide the tibia, rotate
through the required angle, and reunite it. Naturally, orthopaedic surgeons
re not keen to perform such a procedure without good cause.

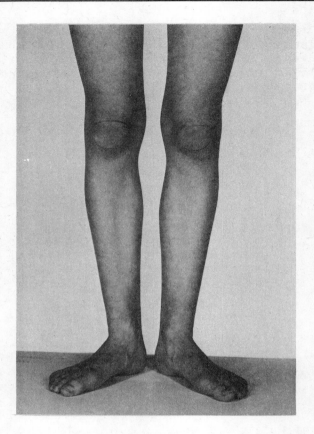

Fig 9.5   Tibial torsion—with patellae facing forwards both feet are rotated outward. (This is the same child as in Figure 9.4—the two moderate deformities tended to cancel each other out.)

Talipes Equinovarus — club foot

A club foot is always present at birth and should have been picked up at the latest by the six-week check. At this stage the normal baby will have a wide range of dorsiflexion at the ankle joint so that the foot can be pushed up until the dorsum almost touches the shin. If the foot normally lies at rest pointing downwards and turned in, and cannot be dorsiflexed to at least 20°, then talipes equinovarus is present and the baby should be referred.

We think it is a mistake at this stage to mention the words club foot, or even talipes, to the mother. Instead you can say that the achilles tendon at the back of the ankle is tight, which does not allow the foot to come up normally. It may be that the orthopaedic surgeon will not consider it to be significant, or he may only wish to strap the foot up. If severe, he may need to consider surgery to release the achilles tendon, transplant the tibialis tendons, or other procedures.

NB There may be an underlying neurological cause, and you should check the reflexes and the back for spina bifida occulta.

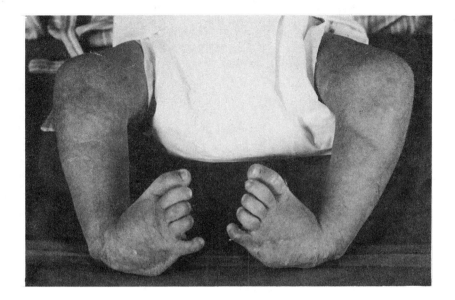

Fig 9.6 Marked talipes equinovarus in a newborn baby

Talipes Calcaneo-Valgus

A calcaneovalgus deformity of the foot is commonly associated with a breech delivery. The foot remains dorsiflexed at rest, but can be stretched down to the horizontal position. The parents should be encouraged to do this passive stretching regularly, and in the vast majority of cases the deformity will have been corrected by the age of six months. Very rarely, there will still be some deformity present after six months, and these children should be referred for an orthopaedic opinion in case there is a congenital abnormality of the bones in the lower leg underlying it.

Metatarsus Varus — Forefoot Adductus

In metatarsus varus there is a curve along the line of the foot so that if you hold the heel pointing forwards you will see that the forefoot is angled inwards. Provided there is a normal range of movement at the ankle (no talipes) and you can passively correct it, the abnormality will improve spontaneously and usually have disappeared by the age of four or five. The parents can help this to take place by putting the child into the wrong shoes, i e. right shoe on left foot and vice versa. However, they should be warned that an awful lot of people will think they have been careless in putting on the shoes the wrong way round, and that it is hardly worth the effort of trying to explain the medical reasoning behind it in the middle of a busy street. They should also discourage the child from lying prone because this aggravates the deformity. If the problem shows no sign of resolving by the time the child has been walking for six months, referral for a specialist opinion may be needed. A few such children do benefit from specially reinforced shoes fitted under a physiotherapist's guidance.

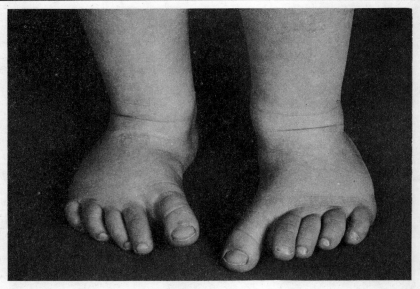

Fig 9.7   Metatarsus varus in both feet

'Flat Feet'

Flat feet must surely be the commonest form of iatrogenic illness. Most of us have a regular trickle of children brought in by their mothers because the child's grandmother was told 40 years ago of the 'dangers of flat feet'. They certainly come top of any orthopaedic surgeons list of unnecessary referrals.

Basically, if the feet are painless and have a normal range of movement, there is nothing wrong with them however flat they may appear. You can easily demonstrate this to the mother by asking the child to stand on tip toe, and a normal arch will then become apparent. You may also be able to reassure her by mentioning the fact that many olympic athletes have 'flat feet', particularly those world famous long distance runners from East Africa who always run in bare feet. Some girls have very lax ankle joints, and tend to roll the feet outwards: this is a nuisance in that it tends to break down and wear their shoes out, but here again the foot is usually completely normal. The mother can buy normal shoes with a fairly strong back and sides, but as these children reach puberty they become less supple and the problem disappears.

Toe-Walking

When young children start to cruise round furniture they frequently walk on their toes and quite a number continue to do so in the early stages of walking alone. This extended position seems to be encouraged by Baby-Bouncers and sit-in Baby Walkers, but these playthings are only actively harmful in the neurologically-damaged child. Persistence of toe-walking beyond toddlerhood needs examination. The commonest way for the problem to present is as a plea for help because the child's shoes wear out on the toes within two or three weeks of purchase!

Causes: *Spastic diplegia* Examination will reveal increased muscle tone, brisk reflexes, upgoing plantar response and presence of clonus in one or both legs. Other features of neurological damage may be found and referral should be to a paediatric neurologist rather than to an orthopaedic department. Treatment consists of physiotherapy, muscle relaxant drugs and, if necessary, surgery at a later date.

Shortened Achilles tendon Examination reveals only limited dorsiflexion of one or both ankles and there is often a family history of this condition. Physiotherapy is again helpful but since surgery may eventually be necessary, it is wisest to refer the child to an orthopaedic surgeon.

Habit This is a common cause of persistent toe-walking. Like most habits, the less attention paid to it, the quicker it will disappear.

Muscular dystrophy is a rare cause of toe-walking. The usual form seen in childhood is Duchenne muscular dystrophy, which occurs in boys (an X-linked recessive). Characteristically, these children have to climb up their legs with their hands to get up from the floor, and they also have bulky calf muscles.

Pes Cavus

Again, this problem tends to be presented as a shoe-complaint, either because the outer borders of the shoes wear very rapidly or because it is almost impossible to buy shoes with a high enough instep. The severity of the condition varies considerably but unless there is pain associated with it, no treatment is necessary, at least not until the child has finished growing. However, examination of the child when he first presents with the problem MUST include a thorough neurological examination since pes cavus is a common symptom of nerve damage from a wide variety of neurological conditions. Obviously, if an abnormality is found, referral is then to a paediatric neurologist rather than to an orthopaedic department. In children with a known neurological defect, pes cavus may be just one of several deformities, but it greatly adds to their frustration in adolescence when they cannot buy fashionable shoes.

DIGITS

Accessory Digits

Extra fingers and toes are quite common and should usually be noticed by the doctor at the examination immediately after birth. In quite a number of cases the problem runs in the family and the parents are neither surprised nor worried by it. Most commonly, an extra digit is merely a small lump of flesh attached to the base of the little finger by a pedicle. These can be very easily removed by a ligature tied as close to the base of the pedicle as possible. The extra digit will then drop off in something under a week.

Where the extra digit is more firmly attached than this, the mother can be reassured that it is almost always possible to remove it with a very good cosmetic result. The child should then be referred to the plastic surgeon some time within the first couple of months, so that the situation can be assessed and the parents can hear what needs to be done and when.

Webbed Fingers and Toes

The majority of cases of webbing involve no underlying bony abnormality and they can therefore be separated comparatively easily by a plastic surgeon. Here again, it is probably helpful if the child can be seen in the first months of life, although most plastic surgeons leave surgery until a bit later. Minor webbing between the toes will of course cause no functional problems, and the parents may well be perfectly happy to leave this untreated.

Curly or Overlapping Toes

There is usually a clear family history which may serve to reassure parents, but, on the other hand, it may increase their desire to correct the oddity (particularly if older relatives have needed surgery to their feet).

Action: (i) After a thorough examination when the deformity is first noticed, leave alone until child is walking well, then re-examine.
(ii) Usually when child's foot is flat on floor the curly or overlapping toes straighten out, in which case no further action is needed. If, however, they still overlie, the toes can then be strapped each morning into a 'better' position. This procedure is of doubtful usefulness but may be effective under a physiotherapist's supervision.
(iii) If there is sufficient deformity to cause painful pressure or callus formation from shoes, then special padding within the shoes may be necessary and even, rarely, surgery, so referral to an orthopaedic department is necessary.

Nail Deformity

During the first year of life, toe nails are so commonly either deformed, or skin-covered, or thickened or brittle that this can be considered normal, and they certainly need no treatment. Infection of the periungual tissues are common in children of all ages but will usually resolve with hot salt-water bathing combined with gently pressing the skin-folds away from the nail.

Thickened nails can be a problem because they are difficult to cut, although usually they can be kept to a reasonable shape by using large nail-clippers and a file. Sometimes it is necessary to refer the parent and child to a chiropodist for a practical lesson in how to do this.

THE LIMPING CHILD

Although this is not normally the province of a child health clinic, you will occasionally be confronted by the problem of a child with a limp. This should never be dismissed lightly, since it almost always indicates significant pathology, and often needs immediate referral to hospital. There are many possible causes, but the commonest and most important are 'irritable hip', Perthes' disease and osteomyelitis. The history may give some clues but the majority of limping children will only have been doing so for a day or two, whatever the cause.

On examination, it is helpful to start by asking the child to point to the site of the pain, but beware because hip disease is often felt in the thigh, or even the knee. Then check the good leg for tenderness and range of movements before turning to the affected leg. Always examine the hips, knees, ankles and feet of both legs and, in particular, compare the hips for the range of rotation and abduction.

(i)   If there is any pain in any of these movements, refer the child directly to the local orthopaedic department the same day, although you may wish to do so via his G P. Also, tell the parents to keep him from weight bearing until he has been seen.

(ii) If there is no pain, but some limitation of movement, you should arrange for him to have an X-ray in the near future, and make sure that the results are seen by yourself or his GP well within a week.

(iii) If there is no pain and normal movements you may reassure the parents, but you should still review the child in about a week if the limp has not disappeared, and at any stage before then if it is getting worse.

10

Developmental Delay or Deviance

An unsatisfactory result of a developmental screening test should be followed by a repeat test between one and four weeks later, preferably by the same examiner. If the result is still unsatisfactory the child should be promptly referred for more detailed assessment by a doctor experienced in this field. Opposite is a flow-chart to illustrate this referral and its possible outcome.

Developmental problems may be presented directly by parents, sometimes voicing their own anxieties or those of concerned friends and relatives. Health visitors and clinic doctors need a very good working knowledge of the range and variety of normal development throughout pre-school years and this is well described in a number of existing books. This chapter is not intended as an easy substitute for these books but as a practical guide for the clinic doctor or health visitor who is not very experienced at judging what action to take when a child's developmental screening results have been unsatisfactory. It is written from our own experience and is intended to clarify when it is safe simply to reassure parents and when referral to a specialist is the wiser course of action.

MOTOR DEVELOPMENT

Early indication of motor difficulties may be picked up at the six-to-eight-week check. The baby may have an overextended back, arms or legs, strongly persistent primitive reflexes, excessively brisk tendon jerks, marked clonus, or asymmetry of limb movements. As a rule of thumb, if only one of these features is present, it is safe to wait until twelve weeks of age and then re-examine the baby. If more than one feature is present, and particularly if the baby is already proving difficult to handle, referral straight away to a paediatrician ensures that early physiotherapy will be instituted. The help that this will give the mother in handling her child may prevent a breakdown in their relationship.

Sitting Alone

Delay in sitting up my be detected at a seven-to-nine-month check, or may be presented by parents. By eight months a baby should be able to sit unsupported at least for a few seconds, and full examination is needed if he cannot. Referral to a developmental paediatrician is required if:

66

FLOW CHART AFTER SCREENING

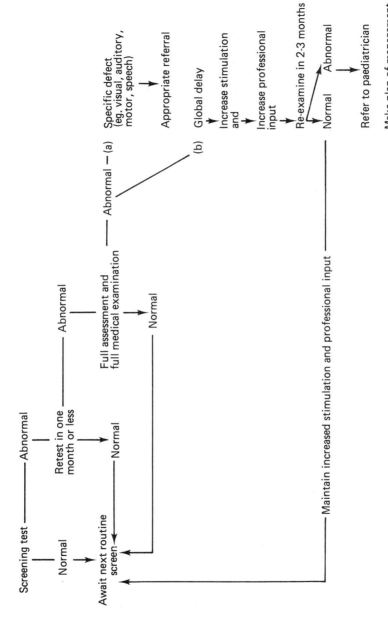

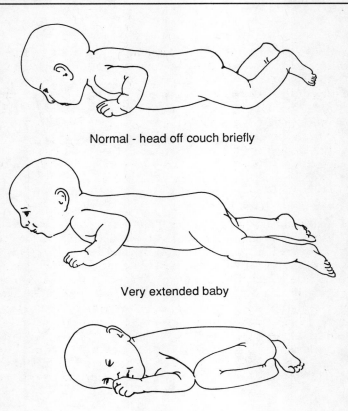

Normal - head off couch briefly

Very extended baby

Very flexed baby

Fig 10.1   Prone position at 6-8 weeks

— any anatomical abnormality is found, eg. of hips or spine;
— the baby's musculature is hypotonic: this may be noticed only as a 'flabby' feel to the limbs and body, or may be much more severe with the baby unable to hold up his head;
— the baby's musculature is hypertonic: this may be slight—tight hip adductors, brisk reflexes, ankle clonus—or severe, with the baby's legs extended like stiff rods or crossing over when he is held vertically;
— other aspects of development are delayed, eg. use of eyes and hands.

If none of these features is present it is reasonable to reassure the parents that he appears to have nothing wrong but that you will examine him again in four to six weeks' time.

Crawling

There is a wide variation in the modes of mobility that young children develop. The majority progress from sitting to crawling but some move around by rolling, or 'commando-crawling' (ie. wriggling on elbows and abdomen) before they can sit, particularly if they are babies who have preferred to lie prone rather than supine. About 10 per cent of children never crawl but shuffle around on their bottoms, propelling themselves by one or both heels, and almost always there is a history that one of their parents did the same. Little significance, therefore, attaches to the method by which a child first gets around but any child who is not moving at all by one year needs full examination and the features that make referral necessary are the same as listed above.

Walking Alone

The range of normality for walking alone spans over a year! Some children walk as early as 10 months, some as late as 24 months. This reflects the complexity of the factors involved in achieving upright balance on two feet – muscle power and tone, nerve supply, growth of bones and joints, balance, vision, height, weight, confidence, encouragement, determination, and so on. However, if a child does not walk alone by 18 months he needs a full examination, since seven per cent of such children do have a neurological abnormality. Some late-walking children have a family history of the same problem (particularly 'shufflers') which is quite reassuring but a full examination is still necessary. Watch the child moving before examining him. Refer him if any of the features listed under 'Sitting Alone' are found. If none are found, parents can be reassured and the child should be examined again if he is not walking in a couple of months.

Later Motor Skills

There is considerable significance in a child who is late in learning the more refined skills of gross motor co-ordination—throwing, kicking, pedalling, hopping, skipping—and the progression of each of these goes in recognised stages continuing well on into school years. Delay in developing this co-ordination can be a great source of difficulty for a child in school but is not often presented as a problem before that. Physiotherapy can be of enormous help to such a child by increasing his awareness of where his body and its various members are in space and restores his confidence in his own ability to control it.

Hearing

Tests of hearing have already been described in Chapter 4 but the following paragraphs outline a plan of action for those children whose results are unsatisfactory.

In the under-two age group the possibility of a child having a hearing loss is more often raised by failed screening tests than by parents. If parents do raise the question, it must be taken very seriously indeed and only when the child has been definitely proved to hear normally should they be reassured.

The action that we believe should be taken if a young child fails a screening test of its hearing is as follows:

— one unsatisfactory test—repeat within 1 to 4 weeks.
— second unsatisfactory test—refer to specified doctor or clinic (whether a local baby clinic or a specialised hearing clinic).

If you are that doctor, you should:
— take a full history, family history and past medical history;
— examine the child and test his general development and vision (since a defect in either will affect a child's ability to respond to a hearing test): if tympanometry is available to you, this should be carried out;
— if any abnormality is found—refer appropriately and arrange further tests of hearing when any other problems have been clarified;
— if no abnormality is found, repeat a full hearing test yourself: if all responses are satisfactory in this the child can be discharged—if not, he should be referred to a specialist in childhood deafness without further delay.

In children aged two or more, a variety of co-operative tests make assessment of hearing easier and these have been described in Chapter 4. All of these are rather crude tests which will only pick up mild degrees of deafness or unilateral deafness if they are done with great attention to detail and every doctor or nurse who carries them out should have proper practical training for this. As with the infant screening test, it is necessary to have a referral procedure similar to that defined above to ensure that every child who may be deaf is not discharged until he has been proved to have normal hearing.

VISION

A child with a squint persisting beyond 12 to 16 weeks of age should be referred to a specialist eye clinic as soon as the problem is noticed, whether it is an obvious squint, present all the time, or one which only shows when the child is tired. If parents or family have not detected it, it should be picked up at the screening test done around seven to nine months of age. A few children develop squints quite suddenly in their toddler years and they need prompt examination. The majority will be only simple squints but all need referral to an eye clinic. From birth onwards, any abnormality of eye movements can indicate a serious problem of vision such as blindness, cataracts or retinoblastoma and it is always better to refer to a specialist clinic than to give uncertain reassurances. Defects of visual acuity can be detected by the various tests described in Chapter 4 and all children who fail such tests should be referred for an ophthalmological opinion.

In some districts all vision screening is carried out by orthoptists (as all dental examinations are done by dentists or dental hygienists) and this puts the matter into its correct perspective of being a very skilled and important task.

COMMUNICATION PROBLEMS

Delay or difficulty with any aspect of development can affect a child's ability to communicate, and inability to communicate can hinder all other aspects of development.

Language development involves both the comprehension of speech and the production of it but is not the only factor involved in communication since gesture, eye contact, facial expression, concentration, memory and ability to make relationships are all involved. Play itself develops from a solitary activity to an experience of communication, and failure to make this progression indicates that a child has a developmental problem. It is therefore important to sort out what a child's real difficulties are when he presents, as he commonly does, with the family's statement that 'He's not talking yet'. A useful procedure to follow is:

— ask what he can say, when he started saying it and who can understand him;
— ask what he can understand (eg. simple commands like 'Fetch Teddy' or complex ones like 'Fetch Mummy's slippers from the cupboard in the bedroom');
— ask about his general development so far and his birth history;
— ask about his family history with regard to speech development;
— examine him fully, including developmental tests, hearing and vision;
— wherever in the examination you have his interest in the toys and pictures you are using, ask him questions to test his understanding of speech, eg. 'Which toy do we drink from?' 'Show me what this is for?' 'Put this on the box, under the table, behind the car, etc.';
— watch and listen to his production of speech sounds and his play.

The average child says more than three words at 18 months, joins words together by the age of two years, and uses complex sentences by the age of five with adult grammar and a vocabulary of 1,500 words. Referral to a speech therapist is needed if he has:

— no single words by two years of age;
— no phrases by 2½ years;
— numerous omissions and substitutions of consonants by 3½ to 4 years;
— delay in total language, comprehension and expression (but requires referral to a developmental paediatrician, too);
— nasal escape, is hoarse or stammers;
— or problems with feeding or dribbling if it is known that he has a neurological problem.

If your attempts to listen to him have been unsuccessful or if you are simply unsure whether he needs to see a speech therapist, then refer him to one for assessment.

If the child does not fall into any of these categories, simply recommend that his language is encouraged by talking to him, regularly reading books with pictures to him, listening to him (whilst ignoring errors of pronunciation) and arranging for him to gain experience of playing with other children. Then review the child about three to six months later.

Even where there is no gross abnormality of speech, a child needs to be able to communicate adequately before he goes to school. Attendance at a playgroup may help this, and may also show up problems. If there are any doubts it is usually better to involve a speech therapist by the age of four years.

GENERALISED DELAY

When a child presents with any of the above problems and your examination suggests that his delay is not specific to one system but is global, he will need to be referred to a paediatrician for investigation of the cause. At the same time, every effort should be made to increase the stimulation that the child receives. Even the most caring and involved parents are usually grateful for skilled advice on how to play with their slowly-developing child, whilst for disinterested parents practical encouragement to play is vitally important. Some examples of how to increase the child's stimulation are:

- health visitor may introduce the Toy Library;
- speech therapists or physiotherapists may teach specific work to do at home;
- playgroup leaders may involve mother and child at the Playgroup or more specialised Opportunity Group;
- a child minder, family support helper or similar person may visit the family to play with the child or to take out siblings so that mother can play with him;
- some districts have a Portage Scheme (or similar early-learning method) in operation which can be introduced to the family and carried out by parents, specialised workers or any of the above field workers;
- other mothers at a Mother-and-Toddler Group may play with their children and include the slower child;
- financial help may be available (such as an Attendance Allowance) to relieve the financial implications of any of the above suggestions.

Re-examination of the child two to three months later will give some indication of the rate of progress he is making. If it is becoming clear that he has a developmental delay which is going to be lasting then the doctors involved must decide who is going to tell the family. All other professionals involved should then be told and a plan of management defined.

Part III

SOCIAL, EMOTIONAL, BEHAVIOURAL PROBLEMS

11

Normal Infant Feeding

Professional training will have taught us a limited amount about feeding infants and toddlers but little of that teaching will be what mothers want to know. If professionals have had children of their own they will be at an advantage here, but care is still needed in exercising their professional judgement. The guiding principle must be to achieve a weight gain which is satisfactory according to the percentile charts, with a happy mother and a contented baby, rather than sticking to pedantic rules. We believe that when these objectives are being met, even with unusual diets, the professional should not interfere.

BREAST FEEDING — 'BREAST IS BEST'

We feel strongly that breast feeding should be realistically encouraged but not over-sold. It is an enormous help to first-time parents to discuss the subject at antenatal classes, particularly when these are organised by the health visitors and midwives who will be supporting the mother after she has had the baby. They should stress that the *advantages of breast feeding* over bottle feeding are modest ones, but real.

1. Breast feeding encourages the essential love-bond between mother and child.
2. Breast milk contains the right constituents for that baby at his various stages of growth, and is sterile.
3. Colostrum is a source of antibodies, and some protection against infection and allergy seems to be derived from it.
4. Breast milk causes the infant gut to colonise with a lactobacillus and the stools are acid, which seems to give more protection against gastrointestinal infection than the gut flora and the less-acid stools produced by artificial milk feeds.
5. There is reduced expense in buying artificial milks, bottles and sterilising kit.
6. It can make feeding quick and easy with no milk to mix or bottles to warm or wash.

There are also some *disadvantages of breast feeding*, and if the mothers have been adequately warned of these during their pregnancy, they will feel less inclined to give up because of minor setbacks during the puerperium.

1. The greatest disadvantage of breast feeding is that it is in fact a technical skill which has to be learnt. Unfortunately, so many mothers bottle fed

75

their babies after the war, that there are now many fewer people in the community at large who can advise the mothers (further details in Chapter 12).

2   While mothers are acquiring the art of breast feeding, they are liable to have some days when the baby does not feed well, and these, of course, occur in the first few weeks with the first baby when the mothers are at their most vulnerable.

3   Although the mother should have some idea how fully her breast has emptied, it is more difficult to know how much the baby has actually taken, compared with a bottle where it is obvious.

4   In a few women the milk genuinely diminishes in quantity, or lactation never becomes properly established, for a variety of reasons.

5   In present-day western society, breasts have become predominantly a sexual attraction and only secondarily a food source, and to many parents there is an embarrassing confusion in their feelings as breasts are bared to suckle a baby. This can be an intolerable embarrassment if they have no privacy at feed times, especially if they are living in rather public households who do not think of this (eg. with husband's family).

BOTTLE FEEDING

It is simplest if the clinic doctor learns about only one or two brands of baby milk (usually those in use at the local maternity hospital) and keeps to these when giving advice, although not to a pedantic extent. Most brands have a special variety for neonates which is highly refined and in content is as near to breast milk as possible. All brands need to be made up exactly as the makers recommend, and most babies require 150 ml/kg body weight/day (or 2½oz/lb body weight/day), divided into five or six feeds. Premature and 'light-for-dates' babies need more milk—180 ml/kg (or 3oz/lb body weight/day) divided into more frequent, smaller feeds because they have a rapid 'catch-up growth' which requires extra nutrition. Some babies demand far more milk than this and some thrive on considerably less. Whether or not this matters depends on one's clinical assessment of the baby—judged by weight gain (plotted on a percentile chart), or appearance, demeanour, and signs and symptoms of illness. It is important to remember that some babies who are truly hungry do not scream for food but lie quietly, giving the misleading impression that they are contented. It is their weight and clinical features that are all-important.

SOLID FOODS

Starting Solids

It seems that even clothing fashions do not change as fast as those in infant feeding; nor are the current clothing fashions defended with quite such crusading fervour as the feeding ones!

The evidence in favour of postponing weaning until after three months of age is well-known and well-documented. Most mothers are now aware of it, although some of them find it difficult to accept, either because they are impatient for the baby to grow up, or because they are anxious to try to gain longer periods of peace between feeds. Due to this trend, we now seldom see babies that are grossly fat, but on the other hand we occasionally find six-month-old babies that are being half-starved by obsessional mothers who have still not started solids. We would suggest that solids should be introduced slightly earlier than at three months where the weight gain is slow, and later for babies who are overweight according to percentile charts. Fortunately, most brands of baby cereal now have a 'first cereal' variety, usually based on rice, containing no protein, no salt and no wheat flour, so that it is rather less necessary to be dogmatic about the correct age for starting these. The mother of a very hungry baby, especially one demanding feeds twice at night, will start cereals anyway, and it is far better in this case to give her 'permission' to do so and explain the need for the solids to be one of the 'first cereals' variety. Nevertheless, for most babies a diet of milk only is nutritionally adequate for the first four months.

Once a child of four months or more has started taking spoon feeds, he can be introduced to a variety of tastes quite rapidly and the choice of liquidised family foods, tinned or powdered foods is entirely up to his mother. The change from milk at every feed to a variety of liquids can go on from this age too, provided there is still an adequate fluid intake.

The change from specially-prepared baby milks to doorstep milk can be made towards the end of the first year (although it must be admitted that some babies have this change thrust upon them much sooner and still thrive). Some babies change to a feeder cup straight from the breast, but the age at which a bottle is finally relinquished may range from eight months to three or four years, depending on management.

VITAMINS

Bottle-fed babies and those that are on baby food do not need vitamin supplements, since these are already added to their diet. Different experts give different opinions on whether vitamin supplements are needed in breast-fed babies. We therefore do not recommend them for Caucasian full-term babies whose mothers are on a good diet, but in correct dosage they will do no harm to any baby where there is doubt. Rickets is known to be more common in coloured babies because they are less able to make vitamin D in their skin when living in our gloomy climate and those from Eastern cultures tend to cover themselves closely with clothing. It seems reasonable, therefore, to suggest that they should be given vitamin supplements, especially during winter months. Premature babies are usually discharged from hospital on iron and vitamins which will be continued for their first year.

FLUORIDE

This subject could be included under a number of subheadings in this book but it is included here only because vitamin drops and fluoride drops are sometimes asked about together by mothers attending clinics. Health education is an important function of a clinic and one which must be carried out at every opportunity that arises, almost by stealth, rather than as a pre-packed lecture on set occasions. Any opening to talk about children's teeth should be utilised and should include diet, tooth cleaning and fluoridation. Unfortunately, fluoridation is not a question that many parents raise spontaneously and, of course, if one lives in an area where fluoride is added to the water supply, there is little more to be said, but for most of us this is not the case. (If you do not know whether your water is fluorinated, you should ring your local water authority and find out.) Mentioning the use of fluoride is now listed as part of the six-to-eight-week check in some areas and mothers are pleasantly interested when it is mentioned. We also particularly stress its importance if we see any child in the three-to-five-year age group with holes in his teeth. These are obviously children at risk of severe caries, and at this age you can at least protect their permanent teeth by advising action.

'Is there any risk from fluoride?' The short answer is 'No'. Some parts of the world naturally have a high level of fluoride in the water, and these areas do not have a raised incidence of any particular diseases. In fact, the only abnormality that is said to have been found with levels in excess of four times the recommended amount, is a grey discolouration of the teeth. Conversely, it should not be forgotten that rotten teeth 'lead to dental abcesses and, in susceptible children, subacute bacterial endocarditis.

'When should we start, how much, and how long?'

Most authorities recommend starting fluoride drops or soluble tablets at 6 months. The dosage is increased at two years and continued until 12 years of age. When fluoride tablets are being given in the very young child, tooth cleaning should be with only a moistened toothbrush, but after one year of age, fluoride toothpaste can be added. In children who are not taking fluoride supplements, tooth cleaning should at least be with plenty of fluoride toothpaste which is swallowed, not spat out.

12

Feeding Problems in Infants

Mothers will often come to the well baby clinic with a specific feeding problem with which they want help. Equally often, their anxieties and worries only come to the surface after gentle questioning, and it is absolutely essential that they should be given the chance to voice their fears. Mothers are never more vulnerable than in the first couple of months with their first baby, so a careful enquiry about feeding must be made at any clinic visit during this time.

GENERAL APPROACH TO PROBLEMS

— Firstly, the baby should be weighed to give a naked weight which is plotted on a percentile chart, if possible with all previous weights.
— Secondly, a full feeding history is needed to find out the number and pattern of feeds, how long they take, and the amount of milk taken.
— Thirdly, you will want to know about the mother herself: whether or not her diet is adequate and contains enough fluids, and whether she gets some rest and family support.
— Finally examine the baby. Heart disease, urinary tract infections, metabolic diseases and mental retardation can be insidious causes of feeding problems.

In summary these come down to:

— *Plot weights* on percentile charts
— *Check feeds*
     — frequency
     — duration
     — amount
     — method
— *Check mother*
     — diet
     — fluids
     — health
     — rest
— *Examine baby*

Communication Between Professionals

It is essential that other professionals involved in helping the mother through a feeding problem should know what recommendations have been made.

79

There is nothing more likely to increase a mother's distress and diminish her confidence in the clinic staff than to receive conflicting advice.

SPECIFIC PROBLEMS

Unsettled Pattern of Feeding

Whether breast or bottle feeding, it is now the fashion to feed the baby to his own hunger timetable. This seems more sensible than feeding him by the clock, and most babies establish a fairly predictable routine. However, there are a few babies who make their mother's day almost unmanageable by demanding feeds every couple of hours through the 24, even though they are gaining weight normally. This may leave both mother and baby exhausted. If you enquire more closely into what is going on, you will usually find that the baby feeds for a few minutes only, and then falls asleep; he is woken up and encouraged to feed a bit more, but in fact only takes about half a normal feed over a period of an hour or even more. Because he wakes so often, he loses interest in the feed as soon as his immediate needs are met and falls asleep, in spite of having only taken a small amount of milk. As a result, he will wake again in an hour or two because he is hungry.

The way out of this vicious circle is to insist on a more structured feeding regime in which the baby gets his feed more quickly and is allowed to rest for longer between feeds. The mother should on no account feed the baby within an hour-and-a-half of the end of the previous feed. If he awakes before that time, he is hungry and will be crying but the mother should be asked to try and keep herself occupied or, if she cannot bear his distress, she should at the most push him around in the pram. In no event should he be allowed to feed for more than thirty minutes and he should then be rapidly changed, winded and put down to sleep, so that the whole operation is over within three-quarters of an hour. Strict adherence to this regime for a couple of days may not be easy but it usually solves the problem.

In the breast-fed baby, a very unsettled pattern may be resolved by mixing breast and bottle feeding for a few days, complementing one or two breast feeds with a small bottle feed, particularly for young babies who are poor feeders and become tired before taking an adequate quantity of milk. The milk in the bottle can be either the mother's expressed milk or a proprietary brand. We would emphasise that this type of complementary feeding is best used only for a short period of a few days to sort out problems and allow a satisfactory pattern of breast feeding to become established.

When breast or bottle-fed infants have been settled and then begin to demand more frequent feeds, the amount given at each feed should be increased: eventually, it will become necessary to introduce solid food, as described in Chapter 11. With a few babies, the introduction of solids can be made before three months of age but this is not really physiologically sound nor desirable.

Feeding on the Breast

When a mother has problems with breast feeding her first baby in the first two weeks, you will often find that it is because he does not fix properly on to the breast. This can only be detected if you watch a feed, when you will see that the baby chews at the nipple. What he should do is take a mouthful of the breast so that a large part of the areola is in his mouth and his tongue is under the nipple (see Fig 12.1): this will enable him to suck properly and his mother's milk to flow freely.

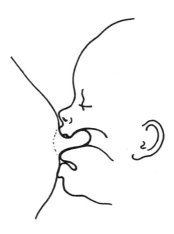

Fig 12.1 Correct positioning of baby's
mouth when breast feeding

Inadequate Milk Supply

Mothers not uncommonly complain that they do not have enough milk. Usually, this can be sorted out by encouragement from the clinic staff and persistence on the part of the mother. Particular points that can be helpful are:

— nutritious diet of about 2,000 calories, even for overweight mothers;
— adequate fluids—not to swamp her, but sufficient to quench her thirst;
— rest—she may feel guilty about this, but she can take it in short stretches during the day if that fits her routine better;
— more frequent feeds—if the baby has only five or six feeds a day these can be increased to between six and eight, which may stimulate more milk flow: he will space the feeds out further as the flow improves;
— complementary feeds may be needed.

Sometimes, a mother will say that she does not have enough milk when, if fact, she means that she does not wish to continue breast feeding. You should try to find out why, but in many cases she will change to the bottle whatever the clinic staff may say, and it is far better to agree to this and give her credit for her achievements up to this stage than to jeopardise your relationship with her by arguing. The changeover from breast to bottle is best done slowly over at least 10 days by replacing one breast feed every other day with milk formula. It is helpful for some mothers to have this written out as a schedule but it does not actually matter in which order the feeds are replaced.

Sore Breasts

Sometimes a breastfeeding mother complains of painful breasts. This may mean any of the following:

The Nipples are Sore. The baby's feeding position and mother's technique of taking him off the breast should be checked. The short-term use of nipple shields during and between feeds may prevent further trouble but a soggy situation can be helped by any of the following means:

— use of a cotton rather than nylon bra;
— use of bra pads without plastic backing;
— using a small plastic tea-strainer (with handle cut off!) to protect nipples inside the bra;
— drying the nipples with a hair dryer after feeds;
— exposure of breasts to the air between feeds (this has its problems in our society and climate!)

Local treatments such as gentle massage with breast milk, proprietary creams and antiseptic sprays are also likely to be tried but are not of proven value, and the latter can cause sensitisation of the skin.

Engorgement If the breasts become overdistended they may be very painful and need good support. Hot or cold compresses may help and analgesics are often necessary. Expression of milk both before and after a feed reduces the engorgement but, if they are too tender to handle before a feed, hot bathing will stimulate milk flow and give relief.

Mastitis and Breast Abscess can be agonisingly painful but sometimes the woman only feels ill and pyrexial with an area of redness on the affected breast. The breasts need good support, and cold compresses may be helpful, as well as analgesics and antibiotics (to cover a staphylococcal infection which is the usual offender). If a large amount of pus has already formed, surgical intervention is needed, but prompt treatment with adequate doses of antibiotic can usually prevent this. There is no need to cease breast feeding and it is important to make sure that the affected breast is emptied as fully as possible, but sometimes the mother feels too ill to continue feeding and then hot bathing and a lactation suppressant may be needed.

The Baby is Vomiting

Any paediatric textbook will list the possible causes and necessary investigations of vomiting in infancy but we are concerned here only with the steps we take to decide which babies need referral for a specialist's opinion and which can be managed with our advice and reassurance.

As already described in the general procedures at the start of this chapter, the baby should be weighed and thoroughly examined and a detailed history of feeding and of the nature, amount and pattern of vomiting taken. In addition, a family history (eg. of renal disorders) should be sought, and a urine test is advisable.

If you find that the baby is clinically dehydrated he will probably need admission to hospital straight away. If he is in any way unwell, the relevant treatment or investigation should be arranged promptly.

If the vomiting is of large amounts and follows most feeds but the baby is not dehydrated or unwell, a test-feed to feel for pyloric stenosis should be arranged. Again this should be dealt with promptly since the baby's condition may deteriorate rapidly.

If everything so far is normal, any further action is based on the percentile chart for weight—an unsatisfactory pattern (see earlier figures) requires further investigation. If the percentile chart shows a satisfactory weight-gain and the baby is well, one can confidently diagnose *possetting*, which is of little importance to him but may cause considerable distress to his family. A few recommendations may help them to cope:

— let the baby sit quietly for 10 to 20 minutes after a feed without vigorous winding efforts: it may help to put him in a suitable baby-chair during this time;
— there are some gel products which thicken feeds but contain no pharmacological ingredient and these may reduce the volume of sickness considerably;
— a series of bibs with plastic linings can be carried around with the baby to protect his clothes, and soda-water is most useful for mopping-up any vomit on adults' clothes, furniture, carpets, and so on, because it reduces the smell;
— one can confidently predict that the sickness will improve a little when the child starts solid foods and will stop completely when he reaches nine or ten months of age.

'Colic'

This is difficult to define because not all babies who cry excessively can possibly have abdominal pains and not all babies who have abdominal pains draw their legs up as one expects. However, it is reasonable to generalise that babies of three months or less who cry for much of the day and night and often cry out suddenly from sleep, or near-sleep, probably have colic.

It is often the case that a vicious circle has been created before you see the baby. For instance:

— if he cries soon after a feed, his family naturally think he is hungry so he may well be overfed;
— if he rejects his milk or falls asleep before the end of a feed, his family will try larger-holed teats, so he may well be windy from gulping;
— if he appears to dislike his milk, his family will naturally change to another brand, often several times, so his feeding will be very disrupted;

— if he cries for much of the day and night, his family will naturally be tired and disappointed with him and his mother may be frankly depressed.

In *assessing* the situation, a good history and examination take time but may be most helpful to the mother in showing her the extent of your concern for her:

— take a detailed feeding history of what milk the baby has had and for how long, of what he has taken in the past 24 hours, how much he has slept in the past 24 hours: ask, too, about teat sizes;
— ask about bowel action and vomiting;
— ask the mother how she assesses her ability to cope with his crying and her tiredness and if she feels disappointed with herself and/or the baby: note her tone of voice and mood (and whether she has a hat pulled firmly over her hair—a sure but undocumented sign of depression);
— plot the baby's weight on a percentile chart;
— examine the baby;
— hold the baby over one's own shoulder or face down on the lap, to see if he quietens; if he does, continue to hold him and see if he suddenly starts to cry again.

If the diagnosis appears to be colic, one then has to decide which of the following suggestions may be helpful for this baby and his mother.

— Do nothing at all except support the mother who is coping well, reminding her that it will all get better soon; and see her again in one or two weeks' time, or earlier (it is not known as three-month colic for nothing).
— Recommend *one* change of feed if not yet tried or one change of teat. There are certainly some babies for whom these changes work, although perhaps only as magical cures?
— Suggest one simple remedy such as gripewater, cool boiled water or camomile (sold in a form suitable for babies by health food shops).
— Arrange for the mother's depression to be treated, if appropriate; and bear in mind the risk of non-accidental injury. Occasionally hospital admission is advisable for the baby.
— Assess the likelihood of this being a cows' milk intolerance (see below) and arrange treatment accordingly.

Colic in Breast-Fed Babies

This is uncommon but is very distressing for a mother since her baby appears to be actively rejecting her. The procedure should be the same as for bottle-fed babies, but there are fewer variables to change: (also see cows' milk intolerance below).

The 'Extended' Baby

This may present as a feeding problem because the baby appears, by throwing back his head, kicking out his legs and crying, to be rejecting his feeds. This aspect of the problem is relatively easily corrected by showing mother how to fix the baby in a flexed position before starting to feed him, and a paediatric physiotherapist may, depending on local availability, be able to make a domiciliary visit to advise the family on handling the baby. There may, of course, be many more problems for the extended baby because of the neurological significance of his tendency to extend.

Cow's Milk Intolerance and Allergy

This is a conglomeration of problems that is not yet fully defined. It includes congenital enzyme deficiencies, secondary milk intolerance following an attack of gastroenteritis, and true allergic reactions: these all tend to be overdiagnosed. The criteria for diagnosis should be: a miserable, colicky baby who is reluctant to feed and has a poor weight gain, usually with loose bowel motions and having a strong family history of atopy. If milk intolerance is seriously suspected, refer to a paediatric department so that an attempt can be made to confirm the diagnosis. For children in whom the problem really is cows milk intolerance, the change to soya milk usually produces a dramatic improvement in the child's weight gain and well-being. At present, soya milk is more expensive than cows milk for babies and this can pose a considerable problem for some families, but it should only be prescribed on an NHS. prescription in the presence of a proven diagnosis of cows milk intolerance.

In breast-fed babies who have colic, there is some slim evidence that removal of cows milk from the mother's diet in some cases leads to an improvement in the baby.

Wind

Some babies clearly do need 'winding' half way through a feed and with experience one can tell when the baby is full of wind—he has a slight frown and pursing of the lips which gives the appearance of a faint blue line round the angles of the mouth. It must be remembered, though, that wind in the intestine is a natural phenomenon and does not necessarily require vigorous efforts at removal.

BOWEL HABITS IN INFANCY

'He has six dirty nappies in a day'
'He only goes once a week'
The frequency of the motions in normal babies varies enormously. The average *breast-fed baby* at three months will produce a motion looking like runny scrambled egg at intervals of anything from every nappy change to once a week. Dark-green stools suggest inadequate milk intake, and bright-green-flecked stools suggest intestinal hurry—usually due to something mother has eaten (eg. acidic drinks, rhubarb, cabbage), but this can be a gastrointestinal infection and the baby needs examining for any sign of dehydration. A reasonable explanation for the 'once a week child' which appeals to the mothers may be that the breast milk is virtually all absorbed with very little residue. However, it should be an indicator to you that baby is at risk of an inadequate milk intake

and his weight should be checked weekly and plotted on a percentile chart so that any drop in his weight gain will be noticed promptly. Frothy loose stools may simply indicate overfeeding, which can usually be elicited in the feeding history.

Bottle-fed babies produce stools of various colours—yellow, brown or whitish-green—and at a frequency of two or three times a day to once in two or three days.

As the child is weaned over the first year, the motions will gradually become more like adult ones and tend to settle to a daily offering.

It should be clear now that it is difficult to define diarrhoea and constipation in infants, since what constitutes a definition in one baby may describe normal bowel activity in another. The following are attempts at definition and, more important, practical guidelines on management.

Diarrhoea

Diarrhoea is a change of bowel habit to more frequent and loose stools than is usual for that child, often with malaise, fever, reduced appetite, crying and possibly other associated features such as vomiting, pain on defaecation, blood in stools.

(a) Take a thorough feeding history, weigh and examine the baby and ask about any recent travel abroad and about acute illness amongst the rest of the family (often a viral respiratory infection in the adults may be associated with diarrhoea in children).

(b) If the baby shows signs of dehydration, it is wisest to arrange hospital admission

(c) If there are other signs of illness, eg. otitis media, or there is reason to suspect an infectious gastroenteritis, arrange for suitable investigations, treatment and follow-up.

(d) Otherwise, recommend stopping milk and solids for 12 to 24 hours and replacing the feeds with a fluid/electrolyte substitute given in small amounts frequently, so that the total amount of fluid intake is greater than normal. Explain clearly how to reintroduce feeds over the following 24 hours, warning that the motions are likely to become dark green, and diminish.

(e) Arrange for the baby to be seen within a day or two and weighed again a week or two after that.

Chronic Diarrhoea

Two important forms of chronic diarrhoea may be seen at a well baby clinic.

Malabsorption. The causes and features of the various malabsorption syndromes are described in paediatric textbooks, but the presenting features may be only frequent, loose or bulky stools in a child with any of the poor weight-gain patterns already illustrated, although in a few children even their weight gain is not particularly poor. Referral for investigation is needed, even though some of them will have no abnormal results and eventually settle down.

Toddler diarrhoea. This is a descriptive label for a condition that probably has several causes. The stools occur two or three times a day, are unformed but not liquid, quite bulky and contain recognisable food fibres (especially sultanas, sweet corn, carrots and meat fibres!) but the child is apparently well, active and of normal weight gain. It is a great practical problem for the family to manage this quantity of faeces in an active child and toilet training is made virtually impossible by it. There is often a history that the problem began with an acute gastrointestinal illness and the cause seems to be an altered intestinal environment, although whether or not this is the result of a change in the flora, mucosa or tolerance of certain substances is uncertain. Management is, as usual, to take a full feeding, medical and family history, to examine the child and keep percentile charts of weight and height. If no indication for further investigation is found there are then a number of actions that you can recommend:

— do nothing at all because the problem will eventually resolve;
— put the child in a disposable nappy underneath his towelling one to reduce the foul washing and antisocial leakage;
— try giving plenty of yoghurt in his diet, which sometimes leads to a dramatic improvement: natural yoghurt is preferable to fruit-filled, but a little honey can be added to improve the taste;
— try reducing the foods known to arrive in his nappy apparently unchanged.

Constipation

Constipation can be defined as a change of bowel habit to infrequent stools which may be of small quantity, hard and pellet-like, or of large amount, dark brown and foul-smelling. When of acute onset it is accompanied by much straining and distress and it may be associated with pain and blood-streaking on the motions. However, in the very young infant with Hirschsprung's disease or with hypothyroidism, constipation cannot be called a change in bowel habit because it may be present from birth.

In the young child, management depends on his clinical state. If there is poor weight gain or the child is not feeding well or seems ill or in pain, further investigation and observation may be required and referral may be necessary. An anal fissure should be treated with frequent warm bathing and a soothing cream, and the baby's fluid increased. The problem should resolve in a few days. Occasionally, a laxative such as lactulose may need to be prescribed.

If there is no clinical abnormality and the baby is bottle-fed, some simple dietary manipulations such as giving extra fluids, a little more sugar in boiled water once a day, or a teaspoonful of squeezed orange juice once or twice a day, is all that is needed. It is sometimes necessary, but not really logical, to try one change of milk brand. In the breast-fed child, dietary manipulations are unnecessary but the possibility of inadequate milk intake must be considered and the baby weighed weekly.

In older children, acute constipation can be caused by a raised temperature, or any cause of mild dehydration, as well as by pathological conditions such as intussusception and hypothyroidism. If there is no apparent cause, the child appears well and no anal fissure is present, dietary manipulation is usually effective but some children will resist all attempts to increase the fruit and fibre content of their diet. A laxative is then required and a bulk-increasing agent, such as lactulose, is preferable.

Intestinal parasites can cause constipation and diarrhoea in children and examination of faeces, plus a Sellotape swab of the anal region should reveal the commoner parasites.

Chronic constipation in an older child is more of a behavioural problem than a feeding one and is dealt with in Chapter 14.

13

General Behaviour and Discipline

A prominent medical philosopher says that paediatricians have no right, either by virtue of training or expertise, to advise parents on their children's behaviour problems. This is a wise warning but professionals who work in children's clinics will time and again be asked by parents for such advice. Perhaps the best way to overcome this dilemma is to allow the parents to tell you about the problem, offer them some clear facts about any particular behaviour, and discuss the various ways which are open to them of managing it. Then they can make their own decisions on how to apply these facts. Professionals who have children of their own will feel at an advantage in discussing behaviour problems, but this is more in their empathy with other parents than necessarily in the wisdom of their advice.

HANDLING IN THE UNDER-FIVES

However chaotic a household may appear to an outsider, if the parents are happy that they are reasonably in control of their children, there is no cause for the clinic to interfere. Where parents come to us complaining that they have lost control, we usually find that they are creating problems in some of the following ways:

— not firm enough
— inconsistent discipline
— disagreement between parents, and between parents and grandparents.
— afraid of being too hard
— afraid of a scene
— trying to use logic and reason with an irrational child
— refusing to use logic with a reasonable child
— afraid to take charge, and in the last resort to say 'because I say so!'
— failing to take disciplinary action with a child before the parents themselves become upset
— failing to praise when good.

CHILDREN—THEIR DIFFERING PERSONALITIES

It often comes as quite a surprise to parents to find that their child has a clear-cut and determined personality, from his very earliest days. It rapidly becomes apparent that some children are extremely determined, and while some appear placid and cheerful, others are very easily upset by quite trivial matters. It is interesting that family order seems to make quite a marked difference, and it is also noticeable that the very bright children are more easily frustrated and are generally more difficult to handle. These observations may be some consolation to sorely-tried parents, but they do not alter the fact that the child they have is one they are going to have to live with.

The Spoilt Child

We all know a grossly-spoilt child when we see one, but some parents seem to be quite unaware of the reasons why their child behaves in this way. To put it bluntly, the spoilt child is one who is accustomed always to getting his own way, and has never been made to consider other people. At playgroup and in school these children will always demand more than their share and cannot accept that other people have a right to an equal share. The result is that they become rapidly unpopular with both their teachers and their peers who soon find their company undesirable. In this way the parents' failure to provide adequate discipline at an early age proves to be grossly unfair to their own child. All children need to know the limits that will be placed on their behaviour, and where these limits are not clearly defined it leads to a feeling of great insecurity and alarm at their own power.

The Defiant Child

Few parents now expect unquestioning obedience from their children at all times, but some parents believe that they have no right to demand obedience at any time. A compromise seems reasonable—that obedience can be demanded over certain issues related to the child's safety and the family's comfort in living together. This really is a matter where doctors are no more qualified to make pronouncements than anyone else but where, again, advice is frequently sought by parents. It seems to us that there are two basic commands which, if not obeyed, can lead to serious danger to a young child, and should therefore be instilled into him as soon as he becomes mobile. These are:

— No (or don't touch)!
— Come here!

If these commands, once understood by the child, are used consistently, (ie. their meaning does not change under protest to 'yes' or 'never mind') but infrequently, they make the basis for parents' control of a child's safety. Thereafter, the control of undesirable behaviour is better done by rewards when it does not occur than by punishment when it does.

GUIDELINES TO DISCIPLINE IN THE UNDER-FIVES

Where parents are having problems in getting their child to behave in an acceptable way, the following suggestions may help them to be consistent.

1   *'Warn once then act'*. In other words if you don't like what your child is doing, either leave him to get on with it or make sure that he stops, but

don't persist in ineffectual nagging, eg. 'If you don't stop doing that you will have to go outside' rather than 'Oh darling, I've asked you lots of times, please do stop doing that'.

It is more important to *take effective action* as soon as it is needed than to worry too much about what that action is. There is nothing wrong with a short sharp smack on the bottom or the hand, provided that (a) it is done before the parent feels really angry, and (b) it is hard enough to make a child cry (ie. is effective). There is no point in smacking a child who merely turns round and grins at you.

Exclusion is more effective than a smack. It is usually enough to put a badly behaved child out of the room which you happen to be in, eg. into the hall. (The child's own bedroom is not a very good place for punishment, since it should be associated with pleasant security.) When you exclude a child, it is a good idea to add 'You can come in again when you feel better', leaving it to the child to return when he feels like it, or 'You can come in again when you are quiet', in which case it is necessary to invite him to come back the minute he is quiet.

This is often a source of friction between parents, and in extreme cases it may actually be helpful for both parents to come and discuss it and agree on a course of action in the presence of the clinic doctor or the health visitor. It may be helpful if they take it in turns to deal with a difficult child rather than always leaving it to one parent.

Rewards. Good behaviour must be rewarded with praise. It should be remembered that for a young child praise from his parents which has been merited is worth more than any number of toys or sweets. Equally, undeserved praise will usually be treated with the contempt that it deserves.

Star Charts

There is nothing magical about these—they are simply a conditioning system based on reward. They can be used for any child from about three-and-a-half years upwards. Any sort of chart will do and the 'stars' can be of any shape or colour or can be drawn in, but it is often necessary to have plain coloured stars or ticks and some red or gold or silver ones. Of course, the sticking on of a star must be given due praise and ceremony. The skill in applying this conditioning system lies in the choice of realistic goals and of suitable rewards. These are worked out thus:

1   Decide on the final achievement of changed behaviour which is desired: two examples could be:
    — achieving dry beds every night;
    — achieving shopping expeditions without temper tantrums.
2   Define how far towards this the child is at present:
    — wet beds every night;
    — temper tantrums in every shop.
3   Work out suitable rewards.
    Generally—for under-5s, praise and hugs;
            —for 5 – 8-year-olds, one sweet or one penny per plain star, two sweets or two pence per gold star;

— for over-8s, save up until, say, Friday night, then choose a reward according to the number of stars earned, eg. 1 means a visit to the shop for a small toy, 5 means a trip to the baths, cinema, etc.

4   Set a small goal which earns a star if achieved, for example:
— aim for one dry night in the first week, two in the second;
— aim for one temper-free visit to one local shop, etc.

5   Check chart after two weeks. If some stars have been achieved, raise goal higher; if none, either lower goal or look for flaws or extraneous circumstances that have caused failure. Gold stars can be awarded for every three consecutive plain stars earned, or some similar bonus.

6   Continue star chart with supervision until desired behaviour has been achieved and maintained for several weeks.

7   If child loses interest in keeping a chart, change the system, eg. from stars to smiling faces drawn by child; or from charts to a collecting box for 'tokens'—coins, cardboard tickets or tiddley-winks.

8   If chart is successful at first but child then stops co-operating (especially happens with older bed-wetters), either use another behaviour method, such as a bed alarm, or reverse the reward system so that deductions are made for every poor response. This is not as satisfactory because it can seem to be punishing failure rather than rewarding success, but it can be effective sometimes.

14

Specific Behaviour Problems

In this chapter we suggest ways which we know to be effective in handling some of the specific problems commonly brought to us by parents. As with everything else in this book, we do not put them forward as the only methods, nor do we claim that they are the best, but they are methods which can work.

With some parents who may be alarmed by a new behaviour in their child it is not necessary to go into as much detail as we have included here—it is sufficient to assure them that the behaviour is normal for that age. The well-known phrase 'It's just a stage' can be quite reassuring; it may be useful to direct them then to one of the many good books written for inexperienced parents of young children. With others, you will know from past experience that they are unlikely to follow any advice which involves effort and organisation on their part, and you are wiser to spend your time trying to arrange some form of separation from their child, for example, by playgroup attendance. For the majority, however, some of the following practical guidelines may well be helpful.

TANTRUMS

'He's got a wicked temper.'

Temper tantrums are a normal response to frustration and are not necessarily limited to early childhood. They start when the child is about one year of age, become more frequent and more dramatic during the second year of life and gradually diminish as the child finds fewer frustrations in his world and better ways of dealing with his rage.

Tantrums should always be handled firmly, although not necessarily fiercely, and when they are a regular occurrence action is needed at the first sign of trouble. Indeed, it is interesting that the child will usually go on causing more and more trouble until action is taken, as if he was demanding the correct discipline.

Parents often ask for advice on managing tantrums, and the actions they can take are as follows.

At the very start of a tantrum it may be possible to *remove the cause of frustration*, for example, when he is unable to fit a square shape into a

93

round hole, find him the square hole; or when another child picks up his toy, find him a different toy in another direction.

If this is impossible, *decide quickly* whether or not to have a battle with him. This will depend on the issue involved (for example, whether or not it relates to his safety) and on the surrounding circumstances (for example, the presence or absence of visitors). *If a battle is thought to be worthwhile*, react by ignoring him, either by staying in the same room but turning one's back or reading the paper, or by walking into another room and, if the tantrum tries to follow, placing a stair-gate across the door (rather than closing a solid door on him).

As soon as he goes quiet, return to him with a smile and friendliness, thus rewarding the *end* of the tantrum.

If a battle is not worthwhile, give in to him immediately.

This gives the child confidence in being allowed to make his own decisions. As an example, he can be allowed to wear torn trousers and wellies to go out without harm, even though clean trousers and shoes were put ready for him.

In older children whose tantrums persist, a star chart to encourage them to hold on to their rage until they are, say, in their own room and then can vent it on a suitable soft toy or bean bag, is often effective.

When a child has frequent tantrums it may be helpful to discuss with the parents whether there may be any underlying cause. For instance, he may be justifiably jealous of a favoured sibling, or he may be unwell. In these circumstances the parents may find there is a dramatic response if they give the child a little bit more attention all to himself each day. Persistence of frequent tantrums beyond four or five years of age indicates a high level of frustration and referral to a child guidance clinic may then be necessary.

The sudden onset of temper tantrums and emotional lability in a previously placid child should alert you to look for a definite cause. Any illness can have this effect and so can any distressing change in circumstances, but a hearing check is a particularly important investigation since sudden deafness is often an unsuspected cause.

OTHER PROBLEMS ASSOCIATED WITH TEMPER TANTRUMS

Breath-Holding. 'He really scares us when he cries'

Breath-holding attacks can be very frightening when witnessed for the first time, but they can be dealt with quite easily. They usually occur in the presence of the parents and start by the child taking an enormous breath. He then holds the breath for what seems like several minutes, and may even continue until he passes out. In fact, if this happens no harm ensues, because at the time when he passes out, normal respiration will take over and he will rapidly recover. However, the parents can prevent this stage ever being reached by prompt action as the child is taking a deep breath. All they need to do is to place a finger in the child's mouth while it is wide open, which causes him to gag and continue breathing normally.

Head-banging

This is common and is not necessarily a problem. It can be related to boredom and frustration (as can any destructive behaviour) but not in every case. It may simply be a repetitive drowsing activity as the child falls asleep or stirs during sleep, in which case some minor padding applied to the cot, bed-head or nearby wall, and perhaps a bracket to screw the cot or bed to the floor or reduce irritating rattles and squeaks, is all that is needed. It can, however, be quite a *severe problem*, occurring many times a day and causing the child to bruise his face and head. There are then several useful actions that can be taken:

— take a history of how the child's day is spent, looking for causes of boredom and frustration;
— examine the child, looking for any cause of pain such as earache or toothache;
— work out with parents ways of relieving the child's boredom and/or frustration;
— recommend, not a fully padded house, which some people try to create, but a legitimate 'head-banging area' of a square of carpet fixed to the floor or wall—the child can be carried to this area each time he starts head-banging and even rewarded for head-banging there: when this has been achieved, progress to rewarding him the minute he stops head-banging.

EXCESSIVE ACTIVITY

Hyperactivity

There is a small group of children who have a clinically recognised condition called 'hyperactivity'. The criteria for considering this diagnosis are:

— activity is continuous, even when given one's full attention: the clinic is a disaster area in seconds!
— concentration span is almost zero, even with new or enjoyed pursuits;
— requires very little sleep—say midnight till 3am—and is not tired the following day;
— signs of neurological abnormality are present.

Such children need referral to a paediatric neurologist and are *not* the subject of this section.

Overactivity. 'He's on the go all the time and I can't get anything done'

Every clinic will have a number of toddlers who are excessively active and whose parents do not know how to cope with them.

Problems leading to overactivity:

1   Boredom. This can apply to a child who has masses of toys as well as to the child who has none if the toys are inappropriate to his age or ability or if he is never shown how to play with them. It can apply to the unusually

bright child if he is not encouraged to discover all that a toy or game can do, or to the extremely slow child who does not know how to mimic the play or activity of others.

Television is particularly boring to a child unless it is in small doses with an adult's explanation.

2   Lack of a place where a child can do as he likes, whether due to a very tidy home, shortage of space or major dangers in every room.

3   Lack of limits to what a child can do, ie. he is allowed to roam from one thing to another with only a background repetition of 'stoppit', 'don't touch' and so on.

4   Lack of physical exercise—not necessarily out-of-doors. Even a very cramped house, flat or bed-sitter can contain a legitimate 'assault course', provided it is supervised for safety.

Useful actions that can be taken:

(a)   Take a detailed account of how the child spends his day and of his sleeping habits.

(b)   Examine him and include an assessment of his hearing, vision, speech and development.

(c)   If some of the above problems (1-4) are present, work out ways in which these can be overcome, keeping to what is practicable for that home. The toy library may be useful for this purpose.

(d)   Consider the possibility of playgroup, activity centre or opportunity group.

(e)   If the parents have already overcome or avoided the above problems, yet the child is still very active, irritable and a poor sleeper, consider the following three possibilities:

(i) He may always be of a restless personality and one of his parents may be just the same.

(ii) He may be a very intelligent child who is frustrated by the physical limitations of his chronological age. An educational psychologist's assessment and advice is useful if it is available, and several helpful books have been written on this subject.

(iii) He may have a food allergy/intolerance. It is unwise to delve into popular literature, which is full of anectdotal 'trials' of diets but no scientific studies. If a relationship between the child's behaviour and certain foods is noticed referral for a consultant's opinion may be the best course. However, many families may have embarked on their own trial of dietary eliminations already and they will benefit from the expert help of a dietician or food allergy clinic. Do not dismiss the family's efforts—there are undoubtedly some children who become much easier to live with when certain products are avoided in their diet.

SLEEP DISTURBANCE 'HE WON'T SLEEP'

'We keep him downstairs until he falls asleep watching the telly at about 11 o'clock then we carry him up to bed, but he always wakes up.'

'He will only sleep in our bed, so my husband has to sleep on the settee.'

'I don't leave him to cry because my husband has to get up early to go to work.'

And so the bedtime battles go on. Sleep problems come up again and again in child health clinics, sometimes as a minor irritation mentioned in passing, sometimes with desperate parents begging in tears for help. Unfortunately, there are no easy answers, but you can help. The first thing to do is to take a full history of what exactly happens and when, and what action each parent takes. This will indicate whether or not the parents are in agreement about the problem and how urgently they need help.

For those parents who are at crisis point, we recommend prescribing something to make the child sleep, while warning them that this will only work for a few days. The number of possible drugs is large and our personal choices are trimeprazine tartrate or chloral hydrate, provided quite large doses are prescribed; or even tricyclic drugs such as imipramine, provided the family can assure one that they will keep them under lock and key. The tricyclics are out of fashion at present, chiefly because they are lethal in overdose, but the fact is that they seem to work slightly better and longer than the others. Whichever drug is used we only prescribe them for a week or two and then tail them off gradually. Some parents will have tried Phenergan Syrup (promethazine) which they can buy over the counter at the chemist, but many of them will say that it is useless for their child.

Having bought a little time, you then need to help the parents to understand some of the underlying causes and how these are aggravating the problem. It is helpful to see the parents again in a week (both of them together, if possible) after they have kept a diary for that period to show exactly when, and for how long, their child is awake. The other point to be made at the first consultation is that some of the parents' actions are almost certainly rewarding the child for waking up, thus ensuring that the problem continues: such actions include playing with him, reading to him, fetching him drinks, or bringing him downstairs to join them. While keeping the diary they can also usefully make a note of anything that they may be doing which, in the long run makes it worthwhile for their child to wake up.

At the second consultation the problems can be more clearly delineated and some possible solutions worked out.

Parents May be Rewarding the Child for Waking Up

If parents sit and play with their child, or allow him to watch television, or give him drinks, they merely encourage his unacceptable behaviour. The older child who complains that he is thirsty can be allowed to go to the bathroom on his own to get himself some water without disturbing anyone else; alternatively, he can have a mug of water by the bedside. These are the only concessions that should be made to requests for drinks.

Child Comes into Parents' Bed

Generally, this seems an unwarranted intrusion on parents' privacy and closeness, except when the child comes in for a cuddle at a reasonable time in the morning. However, if parents do not mind the child sleeping with them in their bed, there is no harm in it.

Attention-Seeking Ploys

Cries of 'I'm hungry' and night feeds after the age of one, should be resisted. It is normal for the body's systems to shut down at night, as we see by the drop in plasma cortisols and other physical changes. Giving food in the middle of the night merely upsets the diurnal rhythm and discourages children from settling down.

Child Has No Experience of Learning to Go to Sleep in His Cot

If the family let him stay downstairs till he falls asleep or if they nurse him or put him in their bed until he is asleep, he will inevitably be cross and worried when he wakes up alone in his cot. He needs to learn that he has a 'sleeping place' and that drowsing to sleep there can be pleasant. This problem has to be tackled by a step-by-step approach as described in B. below.

Some Strategies for Dealing with Crying at Night

Strategy A—Undoubtedly the quickest and most effective method is to leave the child to cry and scream as much as he likes for as long as he likes once one is fairly certain that he only wants attention. This sounds easy, but in fact it is extremely difficult to lie in bed for a couple of hours listening to a child bawling next door. There are some parents who only need the doctor's confirmation that their child 'will not harm himself by screaming' before they feel able to take the firm line they know he needs, and they then rapidly sort out the problem.

Unfortunately, most of the parents who come to the clinic with 'sleep problems' are quite unable to do this, either because they have always given in to their baby and there is no way that they are going to be able to take a tough stand and leave their baby to scream, or because they have other children or neighbours who will not tolerate night-time noise. For those parents who think they may be successful, we would offer the following regime.

1 Put the child to bed at the usual time in the usual way. (It is most helpful to have a set bedtime ritual; for instance, bath or wash, change into night clothes, settle down quietly on bed to be shown a book with pictures or have a story read. This may sound incredibly middle-aged, and middle-class, but children like being read to, and it does set a pattern of winding-down at the end of the day, rather than letting bedtime become a signal for frenzied activity.)

2 Lie him down and tuck him in with cuddly toys, comforters, and so on. Kiss him good night, turn off the lights and leave. There is no point in creeping out and pretending that you have not really gone.

3 If he starts crying on being put to bed, or later in the night, leave him for about five minutes because he may settle.

4   If the crying continues, check that he is clean and dry, and generally all right, so that the crying stops while you are there. Do *not* take him downstairs or into another room. Do *not* give him a drink or food. When you have done this, lie him down again, tuck him in, perhaps without a kiss this time, and leave, saying firmly 'Now go to sleep'.

5   If still crying, leave for ten minutes then return. There is no need to check that he is clean and dry on this occasion. Lie him down firmly, tuck him in and speak sharply so that he knows that you are less than pleased and will stand no nonsense—'Now that's enough. You are to stay lying down.' Then leave.

6   If he is still crying, leave him for twenty minutes then either
     (a) take positive action, by moving him to another room, preferably out of earshot. It may seem hard work but it is worth heaving the cot out to the bathroom or the kitchen. He should then be left indefinitely. At first there will be hysterical screams of fury, but this will usually subside in about half an hour and he will drop off to sleep, secure in the knowledge that he cannot manipulate his parents any further:

or   (b) continue going in to him as in 5 above but at progressively longer intervals—30 minutes then 40 minutes, 50 minutes, and so on. For the first night this is VERY wearing but if one gives in the battle is lost: if one does not give in, the problem resolves very quickly indeed.

Strategy B—Although the above system is rapidly effective, many parents will only feel able to tackle the problem in a manner which does not involve a direct confrontation: for them a step-by-step approach may be appropriate. This will have to be worked out in the light of what they are already doing, but it will probably help if they are seen weekly and a small goal agreed upon each week. For instance, if a young child keeps coming downstairs, the parents may take him back to bed and sit beside the bed for the first week. The next week they could sit further away from the bed, and so on, until he accepts that if he comes downstairs he merely gets taken back to bed again. The same will apply to a child who keeps getting into his parents' bed during the night. With this approach, it is often helpful if the parent who is usually least involved takes the child back to bed and stays with him.

So often when these suggestions are made to the mother of a child with this kind of sleep problem she will say 'Oh, I couldn't ask my husband to do that!'. It is at this point that you have to make it clear to her that, if she and her husband wish to sort out their problems, they must work together and be prepared to inconvenience themselves in the short run for the long-term good of their child. There are no wonder drugs that will bring up their children for them. To make these points effectively, you really have to see the parents together, and on the rare occasions when one partner refuses to come you can be sure that the sleep problem is only a reflection of much deeper marital stresses.

FEEDING PROBLEMS.

'He hardly eats a thing.'
'He just plays with his food.'
'I can't find anything he likes.'

At around one year of age children begin to display their likes and dislikes of food tastes and textures. Some children have much bigger appetites than others and some seem to obtain far more pleasure from meals than others. All parents find that there are days when a child refuses his food which may be because he is unwell, tired, does not like the particular food offered or is just feeling bad-tempered and unco-operative. These normal variations parents usually accept and manage easily. It is when the problem persists that it is brought to a clinic.

Persisting Food Fads or Food Refusal

Occasionally, parents get themselves into a position where their child is living off a lunatic diet which they are too terrified to stop. Examples in our experience have been: sweets and squash at all times of day and absolute refusal of anything else; crisps and ice-cream and nothing else at every meal; and even a child who would eat only dry cornflakes and those only if scattered on the floor under the table! The only way out is to convince parents that their child will eat more suitable food eventually, if given only sensible food and nothing else.

The two essential points about feeding problems are:

1   young children will not voluntarily starve themselves to death or even to ill-health;
2   the feeding problem must cease to be a means of gaining family attention.

Useful Actions That Can be Taken Before Advising on Management

— Take a careful history of the child's food and drink intake over 24 hours, if necessary asking his mother to come back in two or three days' time with a written record of it.
— Examine the child carefully, because recurrent upper respiratory tract infections, urinary tract infection or any chronic illness can cause poor appetite.
— Weigh and measure the child and plot these measurements on a percentile chart, with any previous measurements that may be available.

Occasionally you may find that the weight is falling away from the percentile lines and/or signs of illness are present, in which case the child needs further investigation and may warrant referral to a consultant.

In the majority of cases, the child is lively, with little or no illness, a normal height curve and only slightly lower weight curve. It is then necessary to show the parents the evidence of their child's normal health and growth and beg for calmness at mealtimes. Recommend a change in the day's meals to reduce some of the tension. A suggested plan is as follows:

At Breakfast— continue with whatever the routine is at present without any changes.

At the Main Meal (whether mid-day or evening)—serve the same for the child as for everyone else, cut into strips so that it is recognisable, but in minute quantity—literally, a one-inch strip of meat, two peas, a quarter of a potato and a blob of gravy or sauce to dip the food in (ie. not a puree). A favourite pudding is mentioned but will follow only if the main course has been eaten. Ignore him totally for between five and ten minutes and if nothing has happened, then feed him small mouthfuls of the meal without saying a word and, if possible, whilst talking to someone else. His reward is the promised pudding and a modest amount of praise.

If the child chooses to make a scene when he finds that no-one is taking any notice of him and his food problem, it is best if he is removed from the room and left. After everyone else has finished, he may come back and eat up, or he can starve until the next meal. When this comes, his hunger will solve the problem and he will be the first to finish, therefore winning himself mild praise.

At the Other Meal—do not insist that he sits at the table but make him a picnic and replenish it at intervals. It should be on a tiny plate and consist of little pieces of interesting food such as a small cube of cheese, a finger of bread, a piece of apple, one sweet, and things of that kind. It should be pointed out to parents that there is no need to add extra milk to his diet since this will only diminish his appetite for solid food. Vitamins, too, need not be added, although most mothers with this sort of problem feel happier to continue the infancy vitamin drops.

It is a good idea to weigh the child monthly for a few months and plot these weights on a percentile chart.

Overeating. 'He eats so much we think he might have worms'

This is less common than food refusal and is only a problem if it leads to overweight. It should be seen simply as a bad habit, arising either because the child has nothing more interesting to do than eat or because the whole family have the same habit. You can help in the following ways:

— take a detailed food-intake history;
— plot his height and weight on a chart;
— examine the child thoroughly;
— work out with parents a feeding pattern for the day, suggesting low fat, high fibre snacks rather than abolish snacks completely and recommend that this sort of snack should be taken by all the family and not just the toddler;
— recommend other pleasurable activities for the child to distract him from his main hobby of eating, but which still require his mother's attention being focussed on him;
— weigh him at monthly intervals.

It is quite common for young children to drink excessively and this again is more a pastime than a need. Gradual dilution of his drinks till they are almost water, and distraction to other activities will reduce his interest in drinking. This demands more of his mother's time and attention and that in itself will help to solve the problem.

INCONTINENCE

Toilet training is a normal procedure and is rarely a major problem provided parental expectations of the child, and family expectations of the parents, are reasonable. The essential ingredient is for a mother to deal with training in whatever way feels right to her, without anxiety. If the child becomes distressed by training, it is as well to abandon it for a few weeks and then try again. One source of pressure is that playgroups usually demand that a child is out of nappies in order to attend. The majority of 2½ to 3-year olds are dry and those few who are not can usually remain dry for the two hours they are at playgroup if they are sent wearing trainer pants containing a disposable pad (especially useful are the small stick-on variety sold for women) and a spare pair of pants, even if they are utterly unreliable at home.

Enuresis

Day-time Wetting in Children Aged 3½ or Over. This must always rouse the suspicion of chronic infection and/or anatomical abnormality and an MSU should be sent to the laboratory in every case. X-ray investigation is probably best done by referral to a paediatrician but whilst this appointment is being awaited, or after investigation has proved negative, a star chart can be started. This can help in assessing the severity of the problem, indicating the times of day or week when the problem is worst and, provided the goals are tailored to suit the child, can be therapeutic.

Two examples of the early goals which may be set are:- for a child who never uses the lavatory, stars are awarded for sitting on the lavatory at set intervals, regardless of whether any urine is produced there;
—for a child who is usually dry but forgets to go to the lavatory when engrossed in play, stars are awarded for using the lavatory promptly when reminded to do so by his mother at 2-hourly intervals.

Night-Time Wetting Although most children will become dry at night sometime after their second birthday, at least 10% will still be bed-wetting at the age of five. It more commonly occurs in boys than girls and there is often a strong family history so that the parents are not unduly worried about it. Where the child was dry for a time and has started bed wetting again, it is essential to send a urine specimen to the laboratory for culture.

For children under five or six years old it is inappropriate to start on courses of treatment with tricyclics, buzzer alarms or star charts. However, a simple discussion with the mother may help to improve matters. She should be encouraged not to add to the child's anxiety by complaining bitterly about a wet bed, but should encourage him by praising those occasions where he has had a dry night. She may even like to try simple rewards, for instance offering him small treats if he achieves three dry nights in a row. If he is wet every night without exception, it is better to drop the whole matter and review the situation a year later.

Parents often ask about the advisability of stopping all drinks before bedtime and lifting the child when they go to bed. It seems reasonable to avoid drinks within the last hour before bedtime but although it may seem sensible to lift the child at about 10 or 11pm, in fact parents will often tell you their child is already wet by that time. If, however, they find it helpful there is no reason why they should not continue to do this, but it is more rational that they should wake the child fully so that they do not encourage him to wet in his sleep.

Encopresis

This is puzzling to parents, particularly when their child is reliably dry, and they are often very distressed by it. The problem may have been present for some time before they seek help so the child may also be distressed. Bowel problems also tend to interest the extended family and one example of this was a six-year-old's receipt of a postcard from Grandma on holiday in Majorca, reading simply 'No pooh, no present.'

The Causes of Soiling

Simple Constipation—usually in children who have had a painful anal fissure. They avoid opening their bowels for several days, accumulate hard faecal masses in the rectum and lose the normal 'call to stool'. Loose motions then hurry past these faecal rocks and overflow without the child being able to stop them.

Failure to Become Toilet-Trained. If a child has never learned to recognise the 'call to stool' he will present as never having become clean and is usually called 'defiant'. This is obviously more likely to occur in disrupted households. If he has been taken out of nappies he will defaecate on the floor wherever he is playing and is also likely to show a normal childhood curiosity by playing with the products of his action.

Anatomical Abnormality or Neurological Defect. These are rare causes, having usually been obvious in early life, but of course require referral to a specialist.

Disturbed Mother-Child Relationship with the child visibly hanging-on to his faeces rather than give-in to his Mother by producing them.

You can help in a number of ways:

1   Take a history of toilet training, bowel habits and a description of the present problem and examine the child. It is not always necessary to do a rectal examination since an overloaded colon is usually very obvious abdominally, but it is worth looking at the anus in case an open fissure is present.

2   Arrange for the family to have a supply of a stool-softening agent, either by buying it themselves over the counter or by prescription from their GP.

Write out the dosage instructions in some detail, with a basic dose which is gradually increased until a fairly soft motion is obtained, then reduced until a minimum maintenance dose is found.

There are some children whose colon is so loaded that a more vigorous regime is needed. A child who is that determined to hang on to faeces is manipulating his mother and it is therefore helpful for the mother to carry out the following regime as a means of putting her back in charge of her child's welfare. She will need a supply of oral laxative, suppositories and micro-enemas and instruction on how to use them. The schedule consists of:

— daily lactulose in moderate dosage;
— first day without bowel action add a dose of an oral laxative which stimulates the bowel;
— second day without bowel action use a suppository;
— third day without bowel action use a micro-enema, which is usually very effective.

This is repeated until the child gives up the struggle to hold on to his stools but it is important that it is not carried out in a punitive way and this can be avoided by linking it to rewards for stool production.

3   Start a star chart with the child, keeping the goal which earns him a star down to an achievable level, and explaining it to him in the words that he uses. Supervision of the chart at the clinic is needed at first and as soon as the initial goal (perhaps sitting on the lavatory for a few minutes each day) is achieved, aim higher (for example, producing a stool, however small, in the lavatory each day) until he eventually achieves a daily bowel action in the lavatory at a fairly regular time, with no soiled pants in between. It is sometimes a good idea to turn mother's attention away from her child's bowels by asking her to chart his eating habits while he gets on with his star chart.

4   There will be a few children in whom soiling is just one symptom of many and referral to a consultant is then advisable.

15

Child Abuse and the Protection of Children

Many publications are available on this subject and the DHSS have issued detailed instructions and guidelines on inter-agency co-operation when children are thought to be at risk. All clinics should have access to a book of local procedure to be followed by each discipline when involved in the management of a child who may need protection. Multidisciplinary training courses for field workers are usually available on a regular basis. All of this literature and instruction make it clear that when there is the possibility that a child is being abused, whatever form that abuse may take, the child, and not his parents, becomes the client of first priority and all decisions and actions must be in his interests and not necessarily those of his family. For the family practitioner this can be very hard indeed, and early referral to a paediatrician should be considered so that the child has his own medical advocate.

This chapter is not intended to cover the subject of child abuse fully, only to highlight some points which, in our experience, are particularly important to a clinic doctor. The importance of reading more detailed texts, studying illustrations of significant injuries and attending training courses cannot be over-emphasised. If you can find no local procedural instructions, telephone the Area Director of Social Services and ask for a copy—it is no justification after the event to say that you did not know what procedure you should have followed.

The first essential in recognising a child who is at risk of abuse is to develop your own sensitive alarm systems to rouse your threshold of suspicion. Occasionally you will be wrong, and thereby risk offending innocent parents, but that is a responsibility you must be prepared to take for the sake of those children about whom your suspicion is right and who need protection. There are now well-documented spot signs and highly-significant features that raise the suspicion of abuse and which we list as follows.

SPOT SIGNS

Prenatal

There are a number of indications of a poor-quality relationship between the mother and her unborn child, some of which are:

(a) Failure to attend antenatal clinic.

(b) No response to early foetal movements; apparently oblivious to them.

(c) No attempt to eat suitably, reduce smoking or alcohol, and take iron and vitamins, even when strongly encouraged to do so.

(d) Excessive concern with retaining a good figure and wearing normal clothing.

(e) Failure to make practical preparations for the baby's arrival.

(g) Depression.

At Birth

(a) Lack of interest in the baby after delivery. If this indifference persists after analgesics and sedation have worn off, the prognosis is serious.

(b) Delay in naming the baby (beyond three or four days).

During the First 3 – 6 Months

(a) Holding the baby under one arm (like a cat) or away from the body, like a parcel.

(b) Referring to the baby as 'it'.

(c) Referring to the baby's normal behaviour as deliberate badness or calling him 'naughty' (other than just affectionately as in 'Who's a naughty boy then?'), for example, 'He wouldn't take his bottle so I put him down and then the naughty boy dirtied himself'. The real significance is in the manner of saying this—the baby at risk is not the one with simply a tired, exasperated mother, but with a mother who believes the baby is deliberately annoying her.

(d) Lack of concern about poor weight gain and apparent unawareness of an obviously thin baby.

(e) Lack of care of baby's clothes and nappy area, particularly when this is inappropriate to the parents' appearance and dress.

(f) A baby who is thin but not demanding food—just awake with eyes wide open and frowning slightly. This is similar to the 'frozen watchfulness' of older children who are beyond crying and accept their lot with anxious resignation.

HIGHLY-SIGNIFICANT FEATURES

Failure to Thrive

Whilst the medical causes of this condition must be considered in every underweight child, one of the commonest causes is love-deprivation (probably associated with food deprivation, too). The classical feature is a dramatic rise in weight when the child is removed from home, with a levelling-off again when he returns. The removal from home may be achieved by hospital admission or by a visit to relatives or foster-parents. Height and head circumference also rise during these periods away from home, and growth curves showing these step-like changes are now so well-recognized that they may be accepted in Court as evidence towards authorising the Local Authority to take a child into care. Unfortunately, height and head circumference never fully catch-up and the seriously emotionally-deprived child is of permanently small stature.

Frank Injury

(a) Certain injuries are pathognomonic of child abuse—hand marks, whip marks, cigarette burns, twist-fractures—and photographs or X-rays of these will be found in a number of textbooks.

(b) Fractures in any child under one year of age should be viewed with suspicion, and particularly those in the non-mobile child.

(c) Burns on a non-mobile child; burns on the soles of the feet and the backs of hands.

(d) Scalds on the buttocks or in a 'glove' or 'sock' distribution.

(e) Multiple injuries of different ages, whether fractures, burns, bites, bruises or scratches or a mixture of these.

(f) Bilateral injuries, for example, two black eyes or damaged nails on both hands or both feet, or scalds as in (d).

(g) Delay in seeking treatment for an injury; or presented for treatment by someone other than his parents, because, 'the parents did not seem worried'.

(h) A story that superficially fits the injuries, but on visualising oneself at the scene does not ring true.

(i) A story that is changed on re-telling or differs between historians.

(j) Recurrent minor injuries—conventionally, three such injuries requiring medical attention within 6-12 months should rouse suspicion.

(k) The child's manner—frozen watchfulness or abnormal stoicism.

Before briefly outlining the general procedures that should be followed in the presence of any of these features, two subdivisions of child abuse should be described.

POISONING

This is not a common form of abuse but it may present to any doctor as the so-called Munchausen Syndrome By Proxy in which parents generate medical attention and hospitalisation by faking illness, not of themselves, but of their child or children, sometimes by drugging them. It is usually a diagnosis made only by elimination and by recognition of its repetitive and often dramatic pattern. Such a child will usually have been referred to a hospital paediatrician early on because his parents will have made sure that his symptoms are severe or bizarre enough to warrant this.

In the slightly less outlandish case of straight poisoning of a child with intent to kill him, the clinic doctor is not very likely to be involved, but there are times in either situation when clinic or practice staff know far more about a family and its worrying dynamics than the hospital paediatrician could know. Prompt communication if your suspicions are aroused is a wise course of action, even if it may seem a little melodramatic at the time.

SEXUAL ABUSE

It has become clear in recent years that the sexual abuse of children happens to a far greater extent than we choose to realise and that it is just as difficult to recognise, acknowledge and tackle as any other form of abuse. Books, articles, research papers and working-party reports are appearing in abundance, each one adding a little to the pool of knowledge of the subject but none producing a magically easy way to manage the problem. The best definition is the now well-known one of Kempe: 'The involvement of immature children and adolescents in activities of a sexual nature which they cannot fully comprehend, to which they cannot give full consent and which violate the taboos of social roles in the family and in the community.'

As with the section on general child abuse, we will limit ourselves to a list of suggestive features and those which are highly significant. The subject has so recently come into the open that we do not yet feel able to claim that we can simply describe what we have learnt by experience, since our knowledge of it is still limited to relatively small numbers of cases. In this section only, the cumbersome phraseology '(s)he' and 'her/him' will be used to emphasise that boys may be the victims as well as girls but are less commonly so.

Suggestive Features of Sexual Abuse

(i)   A change in behaviour from a lively girl or boy to a withdrawn, worried-looking child who seems to lose friends and whose school work deteriorates. This really only describes any child with anxiety or depression but it indicates that the cause of that state should be sought.

(ii)   Secondary onset of incontinence, perhaps more likely to be enuresis in a girl and soiling in a boy, but not necessarily so. Again, there may be other causes of these regressive symptoms but questioning of mother and child may produce significant reactions, preferably after you have examined the child and instituted some treatment so that some degree of trust in you is established.

(iii) Vaginal discharge or, more significantly, non-menstrual bleeding.

(iv)   Bite marks on the body.

Highly Significant Features of Sexual Abuse

1   Genital infection.

2   Child tells a friend or adult what is happening to her/him.

3   Sexual awareness in a child, out of step with that of her/his peers and often to an extent which seems attention-seeking or aggressive and is embarrassing to the adults around.

4   On examination   — in girls — a gaping vaginal opening;
                                    — bruising on thighs, buttocks or vulva;
                                    — great distress or extreme nonchalance about the examination.
                        — in boys — a patulous anus;
                                    — bruising on thighs, buttocks perineum or penis.

In general, pre-school children who are sexually abused tend to display:

— overtly sexual behaviour;
— regressive behaviour.

MANAGEMENT

Procedure to be followed in the presence of any of the above signs, and for any form suspected abuse:

(i) Admit to yourself that you are suspicious that this child has a poor love relationship with his parents and that he is being, or is in danger of being, abused by them. Often only one parent is involved in the abuse but the other is a tacit accomplice simply by not protecting the child. It may be impossible to detect which parent is the damaging one but that has little bearing on the medical management (although it does affect enforcement of the law).

(ii) Examine the child, or arrange for him to be examined on any pretext, and plot a percentile growth chart if not already done. Keep accurate records from this minute onwards, if not already doing so.

(iii) Contact immediately all other professionals known to be involved. If your suspicions are founded on only one or two spot signs, the purpose of this contact is to discover if other agencies have concern for the child's safety. Establish communication about the family and try to initiate additional help for the family (whether practical, like baby clothes and samples of food; educational, like teaching them how to play with the baby; or social, like arranging attendance at mother-and-baby groups).

If, however, you suspect that abuse has actually occurred, or if other agencies are worried, too, the purpose of this contact must be to organise an urgent formal 'Child at Risk' conference, usually arranged through Social Services.

(iv) Decide whether or not the child needs to be removed immediately to a place of safety. The simplest way of doing this is by hospital admission, perhaps on the pretext to the parents of arranging for investigations or observation. The statutory procedure for removal is for the Director of Social Services to apply to a magistrate for a Place of Safety Order. The police can also apply for such an Order. Even if the child is in hospital an Order may be necessary to ensure that (s)he stays there in safety.

(v) If possible and relevant, arrange for a skeletal survey to be done.

(vi) Find some means of examining, or at least enquiring about, other children in the family.

(vii) If it is at all possible, discuss with the parents, not accusingly but in order to offer help, what your suspicions are and what you plan to do. This is a wise course of action and can be an enormous relief to parents but it takes an assertive courage that may only come after years of experience. If in doubt, discuss the matter with senior colleagues.

(viii) If a 'Child at Risk' Conference is arranged, give it priority above everything else and attend it with your detailed notes. It is not a fault-finding exercise, nor a bureaucratic over-riding of civil rights, but a means of trying to prevent a child's death or serious injury or lasting damage. It has a clearly-defined decision-making function and it can lay the foundation for effective interdisciplinary protection for the child.

16

Problems of the Child with a Handicapping Condition

The definitive diagnosis that a child has a seriously handicapping condition will usually be made by a hospital specialist. The diagnosis may have a clear-cut label, such as Downs' syndrome, or it may be only a functional description, for example, severe physical or intellectual delay or visual or hearing defect. The suspicion that such a condition exists may first have been aroused at delivery, or the problem may have taken a few weeks or months to develop to the stage that it is detected, but it is the most important function of developmental screening examinations to detect such problems as early as possible. Once the suspicion has been raised, whether by professionals or parents, it is essential that diagnosis should follow as soon as possible, and communication of this diagnosis to the parents, even though this is very painful, must also be prompt. No matter how quickly the process is carried out nor how well the explanations are given, the shattering emotions which engulf a family at this time may take years to overcome.

It is with this period, often very long, from suspicion to diagnosis to acceptance, with which this chapter is particularly concerned. It is all too easy for the family to hide away from contact with normally-developing children, who highlight their own child's problems, or from professionals, who may tell them things they do not want to hear. It is also all too easy for primary care professionals to stay away from the family or make only hurried superficial contacts, not from a lack of sensitivity and care, but from an excess of it, fearing that they will tell the family too much, use the 'wrong' words, or be unable to answer the questions thrown at them. Courageous caring is what the family need during the early weeks after being told of their child's handicap and it may be easier for a professional who feels inexperienced in coping with handicap, to identify with the family by understanding that their emotions are those of grief—grief for the normal child they had expected.

A family may be prevented from isolating itself by encouraging its members to attend a child health clinic and a mother-and-toddler group. This will be hard for them to do at first, but with the support of the health visitor and the company of a friend or neighbour (immediate family are less good at providing this company because they are just as emotionally vulnerable as the mother), the early attempts at integration can be survived and the reward is considerable. Not only will the mother be able to discuss the care and upbringing of her child but she will also be able to talk to other mothers about him and watch him with other children so that, slowly, she may develop a realistic view of him as a healthy baby who has one or more describable problems rather than an ill-defined disaster area. On looking back at this time, some mothers have commented, especially if their child's problem was obvious from birth, that at first they could not look clearly at their child and had only a vague awareness of him as a floppy bundle that cried for food, or as a vast scar (as from a myelomeningocele) that has to be bathed, dressed and fed. It was only when they looked outwards at other babies and saw that their mothers also had difficulty in coping with the normal day-to-day business of caring for a baby that they began to see their child as he really was.

The past ten years have seen the publication of several national reports which make recommendations for the management of handicapped children and their families, all of which emphasise the severity of the distress experienced during the child's early months and years. The reports recognise the value of support given by the family's G.P. and health visitor, but also acknowledge that these primary care workers cannot operate in isolation from the often large number of other professionals also involved. The key to any co-ordination of services must be good communication at all levels. The Court Report defined a new model to facilitate this communication and called it a *District Handicap Team*. It also recommended that each family should have one *named professional* who would work more closely with them than anyone else and to whom the family could turn as a first line of help. Many health authorities have put these recommendations into practice with varying degrees of success, and some have adapted the ideas to suit the needs of their particular district. One such adaptation is used in West Dorset at present which tries to provide a 'package deal' for each family and consists of:

(a) a mini-team of named local fieldworkers, plus the child's parents;
(b) a named team of specialists (including educational specialists);
(c) a co-operation card held by parents to facilitate communication between all involved;
(d) listing in a Special Needs Register which covers all the services provided and is regularly up-dated by all the team members, including parents;
(e) Workshop sessions at intervals for all fieldwork-team members, to increase knowledge of each other's roles, skills and practical problems and thus, it is hoped, boost confidence and morale.

Even a defined fieldwork-team may comprise a daunting number of people for a family to become acquainted with and, in many cases, one member will be chosen as a key worker; this choice can be made by parents and can be changed if circumstances change.

Many health districts now have a *Paediatric Assessment Centre*, which may be as unsophisticated as an outpatient clinic but with various therapists in attendance, or it may be a complex organisation which allows the child and his parents to attend daily (or even live-in) for a whole week whilst he is assessed by every branch of relevant speciality and therapy. Attendance at such

a centre is usually followed-up by full reports of the assessments and som
system of conveying the contents of such reports to the child's family and t
all the professionals known to be involved with them. Nevertheless, it is a
too easy for the specialists at the centre to then feel that everything has bee
done that should be done until the next attendance, and for the primary car
workers to feel that the child's care is entirely in the hands of the specialists
The result to the family may then be that they will receive less attention an
help than they could expect if their child had no handicap at all. The emphasis
therefore, even in the most elaborate assessment centre should be on two-wa
communication, and it is often up to the G.P., health visitor or community chil
health doctor to make the first steps towards this. It seems an obvious poin
to make, but nothing facilitates communication more than the telephone an
a 'phone call to a particular specialist or therapist at the centre may preven
endless misunderstandings or resentments.

The 1981 Education Act is mainly concerned with children who have Specia
Educational Needs because they have some degree of handicapping condition
It defines the procedures to be followed, not only by the local educatio
department, but also by the district health authority's community chil
health department when any child is diagnosed as having such a condition
The purpose of the Act is to ensure that his needs are fully assessed, to allov
his parents adequate say in his education and is generally aimed at benefittin
the child rather than the local education department. However, the statutor
duties it entails can be carried out in a very official, intimidating way and it i
sometimes difficult to avoid this. If the processes of medical and educationa
assessment can be done in the child's own home or local clinic, and if th
personnel involved (whether community child health doctor or educationa
psychologist) are already known to a family's key worker and can be introduce
by her, then the true spirit of the Act may be conveyed.

The key worker or named person for a young child with a handicap will usuall
be the family's health visitor, whatever system of co-ordinating services is prac
tised in a district, or even if no system exists. At any one time a health visito
may have only one or two such children in her case load and may therefor
feel rather inexperienced in such a vulnerable situation. The following checklis
of useful points to be considered may help, but eventually she will be able t
devise a locally-suitable list of her own.

CHECKLIST FOR KEY WORKER FOR A CHILD WITH A SEVERE HANDICAP

1   Who is at present involved with the child? Names of:
 — hospital consultant
 — therapists
 — G.P. and H.V.
 — social workers
 — family aides or care attendants
 — community child health doctor
 — psychologists, educational or clinical

— other professionals
— extended family or close friends.

2 Should someone else be involved?
3 What have the family been told about the handicap?
4 What have they understood about the handicap?
5 Do you need to know more about the condition? (Sources are:- local children's assessment or development centre, social services, library, Help for Health or similar phone-in service).
6 Is the child on the local health department's Special Needs Register (or equivalent)?
7 Are there any useful voluntary bodies available? eg:
— national ones such as R.N.I.B. etc.
— local ones such as toy libraries, equipment libraries etc.
— self-help support/research groups.
8 Would the assistance of the Family Fund (eg. for washing machine, holiday finance, etc.) be helpful?
9 Do the other children in the family need more attention?
10 Is respite care or home care attendant available locally?
11 At age 2
— have the family applied for Attendance Allowance?
— is incontinence provision available locally?
— has the community child health doctor seen the child and advised the education authority?
12 At school entry (which may be at 2-3 years)
— have the parents already visited the school?
— do the school nurse and school doctor know about the child?
— should there be a change of key worker, for example, to teacher or school nurse?

References and Further Reading

Barker M (1985) Enuresis, *Midwife, Health Visitor and Community Nurse*, **21**, 120.

Brooke O G (1983) Supplementary Vit.D in infancy and childhood, *Archives of Disease in Childhood*, **58**, 573.

Curtis Jenkins G & Newton RCF (1981) *The First Year of Life* Edinburgh: Churchill Livingstone.

DHSS (1976) *Fit for the Future: the Court Report*. London: HMSO.

DHSS (1980) *Present-day Practice in Infant Feeding: Report of the Panel on Child Nutrition*. London: HMSO.

DHSS (1981) *Report on Services for Hearing-impaired Children: Advisory Committee on Services for Hearing-impaired People*. London: HMSO.

DHSS (1984) *Immunisation against Infectious Disease: Report of the Joint Committee on Vaccination and Immunisation*. London: HMSO.

DHSS (1986) *Screening for the Detection of Congenital Dislocation of the Hip. London: HMSO.*

Douglas J & Richman N (1984) *Coping with Young Children*. England: Penguin Books.

Douglas J & Richman N (1984) *My Child Won't Sleep*. England: Penguin Books.

Gordan N & McKinlay I (1980) *The Clumsy Child*. Edinburgh: Churchill Livingstone.

Holt K S (1977) *Developmental Paediatrics*. London: Butterworth.

Hull D & Polnay L (1985) *Community Paediatrics*. Edinburgh: Churchill Livingstone.

Illingworth R S (1983) *Development of the Infant and Young Child*. Edinburgh: Churchill Livingstone.

Illingworth R S (1982 third edition) *Basic Developmental Screening: 0-4 years*. Oxford: Blackwell Scientific Publications.

Kempe C H & Helfer R E (1980) *The Battered Child*. University of Chicago Press.

Lee C M (1978) *Child Abuse—a Reader and Sourcebook* England: Open University Press.

Macfarlane J A (1980) *Child Health*. London: Grant McIntyre.

Modell M & Boyd R (1982) *Paediatric Problems in General Practice*. Oxford University Press.

Morgan R (1981) *Childhood Incontinence*. London: Heinemann (published for the Disabled Living Foundation).

Nicoll A & Ross E (1985) Immunisation—reducing the uncertainty. *Health Visitor*, **58**, 285.

Royal College of General Practitioners (1982) *Healthier Children—Thinking Prevention, Report from General Practice 22*, London: RCGP.

Rutter M (1975) *Helping Troubled Children*. England: Penguin Education.

Scowen P (1979) *Feeding Children in the First Year: Report for the H.V.A.* London: Edsall.

Sheridan M (1975) *Children's Developmental Progress from Birth to Five Years*. Windsor: NFER.

Winter G B (1983) Fluorides in the prevention of caries. *Archives of Disease in Childhood*, **58**, 485.

Wood C B S & Walker-Smith J A (1981) *MacKieth's Infant Feeding and Feeding Difficulties*. Edinburgh: Churchill Livingstone.

Useful Addresses

Pre-School Playgroups Association—Alford House, Aveline Street, Wandsworth, London SE11 5DH *01 582 8871.*

National Childbirth Trust—9 Queensborough Terrace, London W23 TB *01 221 3833.*

National Children's Bureau—8 Wakley Street, Islington, London EC1V 7QE *01 278 9441.*

Family Fund—Joseph Rowntree Memorial Trust, PO Box 50, York, N Yorks YO1 1UY *0904 21115.*

British Agencies for Adoption and Fostering—11 Southwark Street, Southwark, London SE11 1RQ *01 407 8800.*

Disabled Living Foundation—380-384 Harrow Road, Hammersmith and Fulham, London W9 2HU *01 289 6111.*

National Council for Special Education—Beaconwood, Borden Hill, Stratford-on-Avon, Warks *021 744 4162.*

British Diabetic Association—10 Queen Anne St London W1 *01 323 1531.*

British Epilepsy Association—Crowthorne House, New Wokingham Road, Wokingham, Berks RG11 3AY *0344 773122.*

Royal National Institute for the Blind—4 Coates Crescent, Edinburgh *031 225 6242.*

Royal National Institute for the Deaf—105 Gower Street, Camden, London WC1E 6AH *01 387 8033.*

Down's Association—3rd. Floor, 4 Oxford Street, London W19 9FL *01 580 0511.*

MENCAP—117/123 Golden Lane, London EC1Y 0RT *01 253 9433.*

Association for Spina Bifida and Hydrocephalus—22 Upper Woburn Place, London WC1H 0EP *01 388 1382.*

National Eczema Society—Tavistock House North, Tavistock Square, London WC1H 9SR *01 388 4097.*

Asthma Society—St. Thomas's Hospital, Lambeth Palace Road, London SE1 7EH *01 261 0110.*

Child Accident Prevention Trust—75 Portland Place, London W1N 3AL *01 636 2545.*

NSPCC—1 Riding House Street, London W1P 8AA *01 580 8812.*

Association for Postnatal Illness—Institute of Obstetrics and Gynaecology, Queen Charlotte's Hospital, Goldhawk Road, London W6 *01 741 5019.*

116

Stillbirth and Perinatal Death Association—15a Christchurch Hill, Camden, London NW3 1JY *01 794 4601*.

Foundation for the Study of Infant Deaths—5th. Floor, 4 Grosvenor Place, London SW1X 7HD *01 235 1721/01 245 9421*.

EQUIPMENT ADDRESSES

Growth charts from Castlemead Publications, Swains Mill, 4A Crane Mead, Ware, Herts SG12 9PY *0920 66411*.

Stycar hearing and vision tests from NFER Publishing Company Ltd, Darville House, 2 Oxford Road East, Windsor, Berks SL4 1DF *07535 58961*.

Kay pictures from P.O. Box 38, Bolton, BL3 3TT.

McCormick Toy Discrimination Test from Dr. B. McCormick, Hearing Services Centre, General Hospital, Nottingham.

Michael Reed Hearing Test Cards from R.N.I.D., 105 Gower St., London WC1E 6AH.

Various vision testing charts from Keeler Ltd., Clewer Hill Rd., Windsor, Berks, SL4 4AA.

Developmental tests from The Test Agency Ltd., Cournswood House, North Dean, High Wycombe, Bucks HP14 4NW.

Index